WARD TWO.

PRACTICAL PROBLEMS
IN RHEUMATOLOGY

PRACTICAL PROBLEMS IN MEDICINE

Practical Problems in Rheumatology

Frank Dudley Hart, MD, FRCP
Consulting Physician, Westminster Hospital

Series Consultant
John Fry, OBE, MD, FRCS, FRCGP

MARTIN DUNITZ

First published in the United Kingdom in 1983
by Martin Dunitz Limited, London
Reprinted 1984
Reprinted 1985

British Library Cataloguing in Publication Data
Hart, Frank Dudley
    Practical problems in rheumatology.–
    (Practical problems in medicine)
    1. Rheumatism
    I. Title   II. Series
    616.7'23   RC927
    ISBN 0-906348-47-1

Designed and phototypeset by Book Ens, Saffron Walden, Essex
Colour separations by Anglia Reproductions, Witham, Essex
Printed and bound in Singapore by Toppan Printing Co (S) Pte Ltd

Contents

Illustrations

Introduction

Rheumatic diseases cover a large part of the body of medicine and affect a very large number of the peoples in the different countries of the world. Physicians who know the rheumatic diseases know a very great deal of medicine. There are some 180 conditions that can qualify as rheumatic disorders, and their differential diagnosis is therefore often difficult – as are their management or treatment. There are relatively few real cures for the different types of chronic arthritis and the management of the more complicated and resistant of these conditions is one of medicine's most difficult problems. The rheumatic diseases make great demands on diagnostician and therapist alike. The twin Saints Cosmos and Damian, both beheaded by the Roman Emperor Diocletian around AD 300, were physician and therapist. Practitioners today have to do the work of both twins. Practical problems in this specialty abound: most practitioners suffer at least one diagnostic headache and probably two therapeutic ones daily.

What follows is aimed to help the baffled diagnostician and assist the confused therapist with some of the more common rheumatic problems.

PART 1: REGIONAL SYNDROMES

1

Pain in the neck

This is a very common symptom in both sexes at most ages and many possible causes have to be considered.

In children and adolescents

Pain may be caused by acutely inflamed cervical glands, often secondary to tonsillitis or quinsy (peritonsillar abscess). Acute painful wry neck may be due to injury, subluxation, strain or possibly a draught of cold air. The neck is often involved in Still's disease (chronic juvenile polyarthritis – see Chapter 11). Neck stiffness and pain may also be a sign of meningitis of any kind, or of cerebral tumour, haemorrhage or abscess. Poliomyelitis must not be forgotten as a possible cause of febrile stiff neck. Any acute fever, particularly in young children and especially if caused by pneumonia, may be accompanied by meningism.

In adults

Pain and stiffness from acute throat infections are less common but injuries, subluxations and degenerative changes in the cervical spine (cervical spondylosis) are more common. There is probably no such thing as a completely normal spine after the age of sixty, and from this time on all X-rays will show some degenerative changes. As in children cerebral and meningeal conditions may cause stiffness and pain in the neck. Tuberculous disease of bone and joint (see Chapter 24) is now relatively rare in developed countries, but not quite so rare in people of Asian stock. Malaria, typhus, arbor virus and other tropical diseases must be considered as causes in tropical countries; some of them, particularly malaria, may be found in recent entrants or re-entrants. Tetanus is also uncommon in developed countries but less uncommon in many other parts of the world.

Rheumatoid arthritis may affect the necks of adults and atlanto-axial subluxation is not infrequent in severe cases. The neck is often affected in ankylosing spondylitis and sometimes in the arthropathies associated with psoriasis and Reiter's disease.

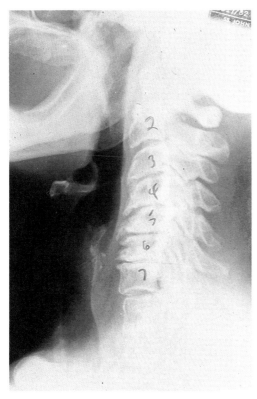

Figure 1 Cervical spondylosis. This X-ray shows the osteoarthrotic changes in the cervical spine of a 78-year-old lady. Degenerative changes extend from C3 to C7 with disc narrowing and considerable distortion of the bodies of C4, 5 and with osteophytosis and loss of the normal spinal curvature.

CERVICAL SPONDYLOSIS

By far the commonest cause of neck pain in adults is cervical spondylosis–degenerative osteoarthrosis of the cervical spine. As people get older:

1. **The ageing cervical discs** tend to narrow.
2. **The true apophyseal joints** posteriorly suffer a similar change.
3. **The foramina** through which the nerves and arteries pass become narrower and may compress or divert them in their courses.
4. **Osteophyte** formation causes further disturbance.

These degenerative changes may start in the middle twenties but are usually more marked at later ages when stiffness and inelasticity make people less able to move their necks normally and more liable to suffer both major and minor injuries. The two most common sites of pain in older spines are at the 5 th–7 th cervical and the 3 rd–5 th lumbar disc levels, areas which are normally mobile but in which movement of stiffening structures increases liability to injury and disc prolapse.

Neck pain in spondylosis

This arises from:

1. **The capsules of joints** which have many nerve endings and are therefore very sensitive to stretching or distortion.
2. **The ligaments and tendons** of the neck which are also sensitive structures that may be stretched or torn by violent movement or overused in trying to compensate for restricted movements in other parts of the neck or upper dorsal spine.
3. **Osteophytes** may divert or compress nerve roots as they enter or leave the spinal canal. They sometimes cause symptoms by pressing on the spinal cord itself.

Common causes

A common cause of aggravation of symptoms in cervical spondylosis is a faulty position in bed, the head being unnaturally angled, usually by too many pillows. Prolonged maintenance of other awkward positions as in writing, typing, reading or even watching television, may also cause aggravation.

TRAUMA

A particularly common injury is the whiplash lesion caused by automobile collision. The body is held by the seat and seat belt but the neck is violently flexed and then extended. This injury usually afflicts the occupants of the front car in a rear-impact collision but can occur in other motor accidents. The risk of suffering it can be greatly reduced by efficient head-supports.

In ankylosing spondylitis the patient's neck may be brittle as well as very stiff and injury may cause such a neck to snap like a long bone, often causing severe damage to the spinal cord, fatal in about 50 per cent of cases.

The gnarled and thickened cervical spine of the osteoarthritic patient is very unlikely to suffer this sort of injury but even moderate trauma may cause long-persisting symptoms.

WHAT TO DO

'Suppling-up' exercises involving movement of the neck will usually produce recovery within a few minutes or an hour or two in acute episodes of stiff painful neck but other treatment is necessary if pain persists.

Complete bed rest is necessary if the pain is very severe. The head is supported on a soft pillow which can be wedged into a V-shape with a bandage. Small soft cushions are placed alongside the head and neck for additional support.

Sedatives and analgesics will be needed to give relaxation and freedom of pain throughout the day and untroubled sleep during the night.

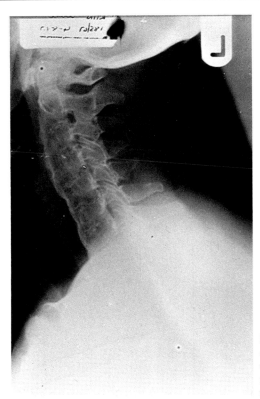

Figure 2 The neck in ankylosing spondylitis showing fusion of several vertebrae and calcification of the longitudinal ligaments virtually converting the cervical spine into a long bone.

Collars   When the pain has abated considerably the patient may be allowed up on the same drug treatment, with the neck supported by a collar. Light supporting collars can be obtained from a department of physical medicine or a medical store. They are usually made of felt enclosed in stockinette but a more rigid collar made of fibreglass or plastazote may be preferred when the patient is ambulant. A very simple collar can be made by folding a newspaper into a strip about 8 cm wide and 46 cm long. This is wrapped in a scarf and tied round the neck, tightly enough to limit movement without causing discomfort. Collars not only support and rest the neck but also keep it warm. Additional warmth can be provided by an electric pad or an ordinary hot-water bottle so long as the skin is protected against excessive heat. Moist heat provided by moist packs is also helpful.

Movement and traction   As the pain abates gentle passive and active movements may begin. In some cases traction may be used at a later stage, the neck being stretched by an experienced doctor or physiotherapist. But traction is a two-edged weapon which may exacerbate symptoms and put the therapeutic clock back. Traction must be done gently and skilfully either by hand or by means of a special apparatus or harness.

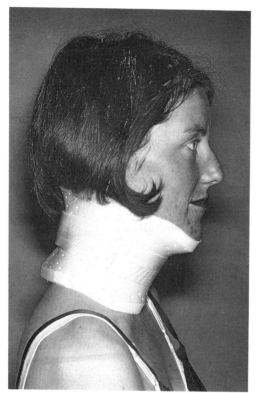

Figure 3   Supporting collar for acute cervical spondylosis.

Manipulation   The same care and skill are needed for manipulation which may be of considerable help once the acute symptoms have settled but occasionally aggravates the condition, even in the best and most experienced hands. Severe neurological complications are sometimes caused by damage to a vertebral artery and adhesions of cord and nerve roots may render them liable to injury by sudden or forcible movements. Manipulation or uncontrolled movement under anaesthesia may aggravate symptoms or cause serious damage, as may any sudden or unexpected movement of the head. Traction or manipulation should always be preceded by X-ray examination.

PRACTICAL POINTS

● Acute pain in neck in children is most often due to inflamed neck glands or acute wry neck.
● In adults degenerative cervical spondylosis is the most usual cause.
● Cervical spondylosis is managed by rest, collar, and analgesics.
● Beware of inexperienced or amateur traction and manipulation.

2

The shoulder

The term 'frozen shoulder' is often used when the joint is not truly 'frozen' by stiffness but too painful to be put through its full range of movements. If this is due to rheumatoid arthritis there will be signs in other joints: monarticular rheumatoid arthritis is rare and rheumatoid arthritis confined to one shoulder is very rare indeed. In polymyalgia rheumatica both shoulders are stiff in the early morning and improve as the day goes on; the hips may be similarly affected but other joints are rarely involved. While the glenohumeral joint is often attacked by the inflammatory arthropathies it is seldom affected by degenerative changes unless it has been dislocated or injured in the past. The acromioclavicular joint is more likely to be affected by osteoarthrosis.

When one shoulder is the only painful joint the trouble is more likely to be around the joint than in it. The condition is one of periarthritis rather than arthritis. Neck pain is usually referred laterally and the pain caused by cervical spondylosis, a very common condition (see Chapter 1), is often felt in the shoulder. In such cases movements of the neck are stiff and painful but the shoulder can move freely if the neck is completely immobilized. Pain may also be referred to the shoulder from disease in the chest or upper abdomen.

Causes of pain in the shoulder

- Periarthritis
- Referred neck pain
- Rheumatoid arthritis
- Polymyalgia rheumatica
- Inflammatory arthropathy in the glenohumeral joint
- Osteoarthrosis in the acromioclavicular joint
- Disease in the chest or upper abdomen

ANATOMY

The anatomy of the shoulder is complicated. It is a highly mobile joint built for movement rather than stability and has four separate mechanisms: glenohumeral,

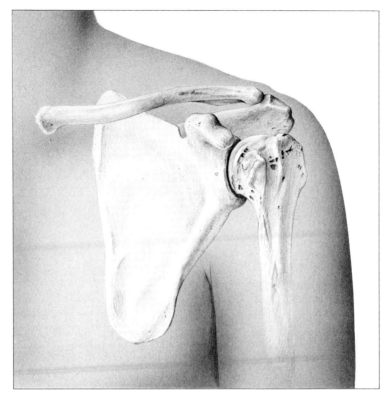

Figure 4   The anatomy of the shoulder.

sternoclavicular and acromioclavicular joint movements and movement of the scapula on the thoracic wall. The glenohumeral joint is surrounded by the rotator cuff which consists of the tendons of supraspinatus, infraspinatus, teres minor and subscapularis. The subacromial (subdeltoid) bursa separates this rotator cuff from the coracodeltoid arch and deltoid muscles.

SYNDROMES

Supraspinatus syndrome

Rupture or injury of the supraspinatus tendon may follow a fall on the outstretched hand, a sprain or a period of unaccustomed use. The arm cannot be abducted and attempted movement is painful. There is pain on resisted abduction. Partial rupture or milder injury causes less weakness but there is pain referred to the point of the shoulder on partial abduction.

Calcification may occur in the muscle near its insertion and is seen in X-rays as a small opacity, usually only a few millimetres in diameter, between the acromion process and the humerus. Such calcific deposits in or on the tendon may be apparently primary or they may appear in areas of degenerative tendinitis. Larger deposits, 5 mm or more in diameter, may cause pain on movement of the arm and may burst into the subacromial bursa where they cause severe pain even at rest.

Treatment   Surgical drainage is needed in some cases but most settle down with rest and analgesics, possibly with the help of injections of a local anaesthetic or corticosteroids (see Chapters 30 and 31). There are only three synovial spaces in the shoulder: the glenohumeral and acromioclavicular joints and the subacromial bursa. Any injections elsewhere must go into the tissues themselves and an injection into a tendon may cause it to rupture. Pain due to a tear of the supraspinatus may be relieved temporarily by injecting local anaesthetic into the area between the acromion process and the head of the humerus.

Subacromial bursitis

This may occur in association with a supraspinatus lesion. X-rays are usually normal but in a minority of cases they show calcified deposits in or on the surface of the tendon. Subacromial bursitis may also occur in rheumatoid arthritis or as a result of infection or for no ascertainable reason.

Causes of pain   Bursitis alone is rarely the sole cause of the pain. The part played by calcific tendinous deposits is doubted by some workers while others believe that deposits of hydroxyapatite at the site of injury act as local irritants and may burst into the bursa where they cause inflammation and pain. It is not normal for the subacromial bursa to communicate with the glenohumeral joint but arthrographic studies show that communication does occur sometimes and is quite common in cases of supraspinatus tendinitis.

   During normal movement of the shoulder upwards and outwards in abduction of the arm, the rotator cuff tendons, particularly that of supraspinatus, pass under the coracoacromial arch. Because the arch is narrow and low any abnormality or swelling of the tendon may cause pain on abduction. Pain begins when the arm approaches a right-angled abduction from the body (45°–125°).

   In rheumatoid arthritis much of the swelling and some of the discomfort is caused by involvement of the bursa rather than of the glenohumeral joint with which it may communicate.

Treatment   Rapid relief from the pain of subacromial bursitis is usually obtained by injection into the bursa of a local anaesthetic with a corticosteroid (eg, 3–5 ml of lignocaine with 20 mg of hydrocortisone).

Biceps tendinitis

The tendon of the long head of biceps runs in a sleeve-like synovial extension of the shoulder joint in a groove on the anterior surface of the humerus. Here it is exposed to mechanical strain by which it may be injured or ruptured. Tenderness is greatest in the bicipital groove but may also occur at the distal insertion of the biceps in the cubital fossa. Kozin[1] notes that, in addition to tendinitis, tenosynovitis or rupture, the bicipital tendon may become lengthened by friction and inflammation. It may also be subluxated or dislocated from the intertubercular groove in which it lies.

Treatment   A recently ruptured tendon in a young person should be repaired surgically but if several weeks have passed, or if the patient is elderly, conservative treatment may be preferred. A slipping tendon may need surgical fixation.

'Frozen shoulder'

'Frozen shoulder' or adhesive capsulitis often proves to be painful as well as stiff but in the absence of arthritis it usually returns to complete normality even if it often takes one to two years to do so. This is a condition in which there is capsulitis but little or no synovitis, and the outcome is quite different from that of a rheumatoid involvement of the joint which quite often results in permanent stiffness.

Adhesive capsulitis lasts many months, during which it causes considerable pain, disability, demoralization and loss of sleep. The pain is often worse at night and it is painful to lie on the affected shoulder. X-rays remain normal unless there is some degree of disuse osteoporosis.

Treatment   This is a condition in which recovery is likely to be delayed by overuse of the shoulder or any attempt at vigorous exercise. In the early and more painful stage the arm must be kept in a sling and analgesics and anti-inflammatory agents are needed. A more positive programme of gentle exercises, injections and possibly manipulation only becomes permissible several months after the onset and when there has been a considerable abatement of symptoms.

It has been suggested that capsulitis may be due to a sympathetic nerve disorder (see the following section: The shoulder-hand syndrome). Some workers[2] think that stiff, painful shoulders do best with one to three paired injections of lignocaine and 20 mg of either methylprednisolone or triamcinolone acetonide given at weekly intervals into both the glenohumeral joint and the subcoracoid bursa. Injection into only one of these sites rarely produces adequate relief of symptoms.

The shoulder-hand (Steinbrocker) syndrome[3,4]

This rare condition seems to be due to an autonomic nerve disorder which may follow a stroke, herpes zoster, a myocardial infarct or injuries or burns of the shoulder or arm. A few weeks after the precipitating condition the patient develops pain in the hand and shoulder. The hand is hot, swollen and sweaty at first, and all movements are very restricted. At onset the shoulder is painful and becomes stiff as the pain abates. Muscle atrophy and stiffness follow, the limb becoming stiff, wasted, tender and useless. X-rays show only a patchy osteoporosis of the hand and the head of the humerus.

In many cases no cause for the condition can be found. There have been rare associations with phenobarbitone or isoniazid therapy. The shoulder condition appears to be a capsulitis, possibly related to the adhesive capsulitis described previously. The type of capsulitis seen in these two conditions appears to be confined to the shoulder. It is usually unilateral but sometimes affects both shoulders.

Treatment   The majority of cases are mild and in these there is complete recovery within three to twenty-four months, but those who are seriously affected may remain so for the rest of their lives. Some patients are helped by cervical sympathectomy, and some by high doses of corticosteroid: 60–80 mg of prednisolone daily for two to three weeks followed by gradual reduction.

Acromioclavicular arthritis

This is usually traumatic or degenerative and is relatively more common in sportspeople.[5] It should be treated with rest and support. Intra-articular injections of local anaesthetic with corticosteroid can be used if symptoms are severe.

Malignant disease

This may cause pain in the shoulder. Primary tumours, usually bronchial carcinomata, may cause pain and muscle wasting of the shoulder, as may basal pleurisy, aortic aneurysm or pericarditis. Lesions of the liver, gall bladder or pancreas may cause pain referred to the right shoulder. The breast and prostate are the most common sources of metastases into the bones of this joint.

Endocrine disorders

Shoulder pain has been reported as occurring in diabetes mellitus,[6] although this is rare in my experience and with hyper-[7] and hypothryoidism.[8,9]

WHAT TO DO

Apart from true arthritis affecting the glenohumeral joint, the aetiological background and the pathology of the peri-articular, bursal and tendinous lesions is somewhat obscure, with bursitis and tendinous lesions overlapping and capsulitis taking various forms. Treatment is therefore empirical rather than scientific.

Injections

Results of local injections are highly variable – some being helpful, many useless and a few harmful – much depending on exactly what condition is present in the tissues and into exactly which tissue the injected material is put.

   They may cause rupture of tendons, either by their own traumatic effect on a weakened tendon or by allowing overuse when pain has been suppressed.

Capsulitis

In either of the forms of this condition that have been mentioned vigorous physical treatment does more harm than good in the early stages and injections may be useless or even harmful. The patient is likely to do himself less damage than might be done by enthusiastic manipulators or physiotherapists because the acute pain of the early stages will restrain him from being too active at this time.

The acute painful shoulder

During the acute stage of a calcific bursitis the area is so painful, swollen and hot that sepsis may be suspected and the presence of more than slight fever may reinforce this suspicion. In such cases the joint should be aspirated, but the fluid may be too thick to pass through any needle and surgical drainage may be necessary. Happily this is seldom needed and the condition often settles within a few days on conservative treatment. In persistent cases of shoulder pain arthrography may help in deciding what is going on in the tissues and what therapy is needed.

The acute painful shoulder remains something of an enigma as is apparent from the different accounts given by different authors and the different therapies that they advise. Rest with the arm in a sling seems to be the logical treatment for acute and very painful bursitis or tendinitis and in the early stages of capsulitis as well as for any very painful shoulder for which a firm diagnosis has not yet been made. It has been suggested but not proved that enforced immobility contributes to the development of some cases of shoulder-hand syndrome. If we definitely knew this to be true, early mobilization would be the correct treatment.

One thing that does seem to be true of the conditions described is that most of them recover completely or almost completely if they are given enough time. Emergency or surgical measures are therefore best reserved for those septic or traumatic lesions that evidently need them.

PRACTICAL POINTS

- Shoulder pain can result from a wide variety of syndromes:
  —Supraspinatus syndrome
  —Subacromial bursitis
  —Biceps tendinitis
  —Adhesive capsulitis ('frozen shoulder')
  —The shoulder-hand (Steinbrocker) syndrome
  —Acromioclavicular arthritis
  —Malignant disease
  —Endocrine disorders
- Rest with arm in a sling is correct treatment until a diagnosis has been made.
- Arthography may be useful in determining the correct therapy for persistent shoulder pain.
- Results of injection treatment are variable, and may include rupture of tendons.
- Injections, manipulation and physiotherapy are all contraindicated in the early stages of capsulitis.
- Most conditions recover in time – so avoid surgery wherever possible.

3

Reading the hand

Long experience as an examiner for qualifying degrees and higher diplomas has taught me that the candidate who can read the clues offered by a patient's hands is usually one who has a sound basic knowledge of clinical medicine. The hand that opens my door and offers me the referral letter frequently offers me a valuable pointer to the diagnosis and sometimes presents it on a plate even before the letter has been opened or a word of medical history spoken. Few parts of the human body are as informative as the hand and few can tell you as much by their general appearance and the way they function. This is particularly true of hands affected by rheumatic disease.

THE GENERAL GROUPS OF RHEUMATIC DISEASE IN THE HANDS

Osteoarthrosis

The gnarled or knobbly hand of osteoarthrosis is often the product of hard and prolonged manual work and may be part of a generalized osteoarthrosis. In Europe it is most common in white women at or after the end of their child-bearing life. These women are often poor or very poor and have been forced to bear the curse of Adam as well as the curse of Eve. However, osteoarthrotic knobbly hands also occur in people of all classes and all occupations.

Osteoarthrosis may be confined to the hand in the case of certain occupations which involve repeated hand trauma. Sufferers include professional wicket-keepers and baseball catchers. There may be a family proclivity to what is sometimes called 'wear-and-tear arthritis' but there are also family proclivities to grinding poverty and such hand-battering trades as keeping wicket.

The joints most frequently involved in osteoarthrosis of the hands are the terminal interphalangeals (causing Heberden's nodes) and the carpometacarpals at the bases of the thumbs. The proximal interphalangeal joints are sometimes affected (Bouchard's nodes). A patchy distribution of osteoarthrosis in metacarpophalangeal, wrist or

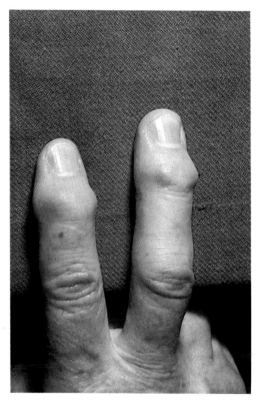

Figure 5   Heberden's bony nodes in an osteoarthrotic hand. The proximal interphalangeal joint of the middle finger is also affected (Bouchard's node).

intercarpal articulations suggests that trauma may be the cause. A diffuse distribution suggests pre-existing inflammatory polyarthritis affecting all finger joints and wrists.

There are usually no signs of inflammation in an osteoarthrotic hand but when a terminal interphalangeal joint is first affected in generalized menopausal osteo-arthrosis it may be tender and red. This 'hot Heberden's node' may show a small vesicle which can be punctured with a needle to release a minute bead of viscous fluid containing hyaluronic acid from degenerating cartilage.

Rheumatoid

The inflamed hand may be a result of septic infection or, rarely, of true gout. In such cases it is tender, red and swollen, and inflammation is usually confined to one area.

In rheumatoid arthritis the terminal interphalangeal joints are usually spared but the wrists, metacarpophalangeal and proximal interphalangeal joints tend to be

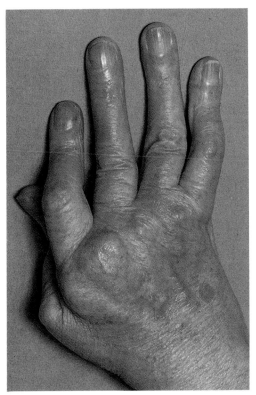

Figure 6 Typical advanced rheumatoid arthritis with ulnar deviation.

affected symmetrically and bilaterally. The swollen joints are tender and lateral pressure over the proximal interphalangeal joints is more painful than antero-posterior pressure. When the hand is half clenched the hollows between knuckles are obliterated. The normal shape of the wrist is lost. There is often pain on pressure over wrists, knuckles and ulnar styloids which may be prominent and abnormally compressible.

The joints are stiff and painful to move. The strength of the grip is greatly reduced and the patient may be unable to make a tight fist or press the finger-nails into the palm of the hand. Fluid may be palpable in the joints and/or synovial sheaths. Although rheumatoid arthritis is an inflammatory condition the hands are often cold, pale and clammy with pink palms and fingertips.

The seronegative arthropathies   In these a similar appearance may be seen, but in psoriatic arthritis the terminal interphalangeal joints are often affected and the

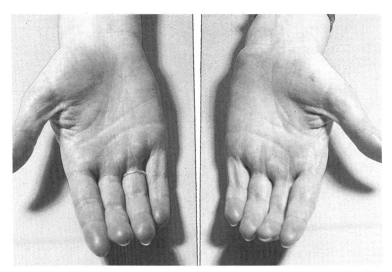

Figure 7   Intrinsic muscle wasting in hands due to median nerve compression in the carpal tunnel.

finger-nails usually show rigidity, pitting or yellow discoloration. The terminal interphalangeal joints may also be tender and swollen in juvenile chronic polyarthritis (Still's disease) which usually remains seronegative and is not a form of rheumatoid arthritis. Other seronegative arthropathies include those associated with colitis and rubella; neither of these is likely to lead to persistent or permanent changes. Systemic lupus erythematosus may produce similar changes in the hands and they are sometimes, if rarely, found in polyarteritis nodosa.

Neurological

The wasted hand   If there is wasting of the intrinsic muscles of the hand its cause will usually be found in the central nervous system or a peripheral nerve; but wasting without sensory deficit may be due to prolonged immobility from any cause, including osteoarthritis and polyarthritis.

Skin-connective tissues

The contracted hand   In scleroderma (progressive systemic sclerosis) the skin is tight over the whole hand – the fingers being pinched, contracted and bent and sometimes having scars over their tips where the terminal phalanges and their surrounding tissues are foreshortened.

In Sudek's atrophy following trauma there are atrophic changes in bone and soft tissues. There are similar atrophic changes in the 'shoulder-hand syndrome' of Steinbrocker (see Chapter 2) which follows injury to the shoulder or, sometimes, coronary thrombosis, the skin of the hand becoming shiny and smooth and its muscles atrophied.

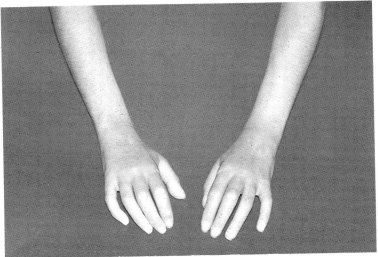

Figure 8 Contracted hands and forearms of scleroderma (progressive systemic sclerosis).

There may be joint swelling in the early stages of scleroderma and this may suggest rheumatoid arthritis before it gives way to the typical sclerodermatous changes. Puffy swelling of the hand may occur as a first stage of the shoulder-hand syndrome.

Oedema

The puffy, noninflamed hand may be due to venous obstruction as after breast resection for malignancy or after thrombosis of arm veins. It may also be caused by lymphatic obstruction due to carcinoma of the breast, filariasis or, rarely, rheumatoid arthritis.

The thickened hand As the hand grows older the fingers may become slightly thicker so that rings are found to be tighter and more difficult to remove. In acromegaly the fingers become spatulate and the whole hand thickens. Thickening and clubbing of the fingers with laying down of periosteal new bone occurs in pseudohypertrophic pulmonary osteoarthropathy, a condition usually but not invariably associated with a neoplasm, most commonly carcinoma of the lung.

Nodes and effusions

Lumps on the hand may be:

1. **Bony nodes** as in the Heberden's nodes of terminal interphalangeal joints.
2. **Rheumatoid nodules.**

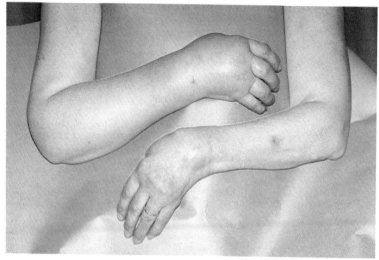

Figure 9 Oedematous right hand and forearm due to lymphatic obstruction (lymphoedema) in rheumatoid arthritis, an uncommon finding. Rheumatoid changes without lymphoedema are seen in the left hand.

Figure 10 Bony Heberden's and Bouchard's nodes in osteoarthrotic hands with traumatic distortion of the right middle finger.

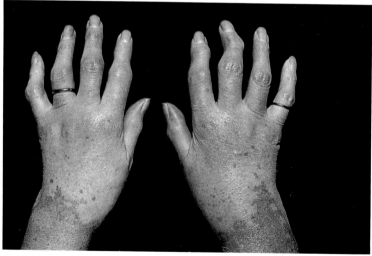

3. **Innocent fatty-fibrous nodes** over the dorsal surfaces of the proximal interphalangeal joints (Garrod's fatty pads or Hale-White's nodes).
4. **Localized synovial swellings** from which the fluid can be pressed back into the joint. These are often seen in rheumatoid arthritis.

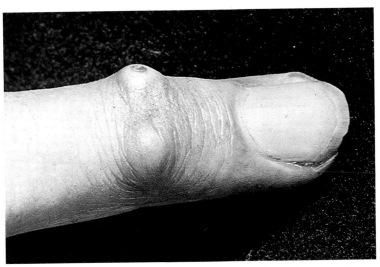

Figure 11   Rheumatoid nodules masquerading as Heberden's nodes. They are soft, not bony, and appear at points of friction and contact with hard surfaces. A small vascular rheumatoid lesion is present in one. These 'pseudo-Heberden's' rheumatoid nodes are uncommon and may cause diagnostic confusion.

Figure 12   Hale-White's nodes (Garrod's fatty pads) over the backs of the proximal interphalangeal joints are not a manifestation of disease, cause no discomfort and are only of cosmetic and diagnostic importance as they may be confused with rheumatoid nodules.

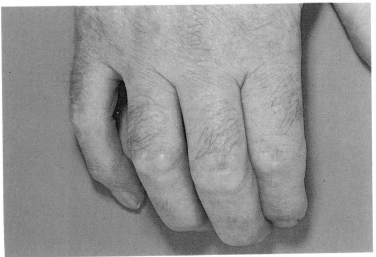

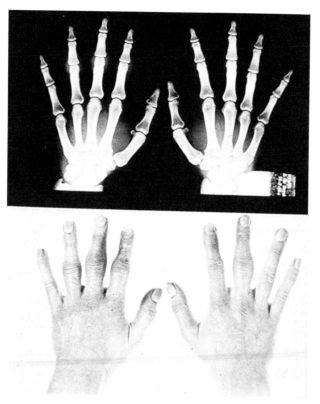

Figure 13   Synovial swelling of the proximal interphalangeal joints in early rheumatoid arthritis. They are due to inflammatory changes and are tender to pressure. No obvious X-ray changes are present at this early stage except periarthrodal osteoporosis.

5. **Localized tenosynovial effusions,** as in extensor or flexor digital sheaths or the extensor communis sheath on the back of the hand, are all common manifestations of rheumatoid arthritis. Ordinary wrist ganglia are firmer in consistency. They may be found in patients with rheumatoid arthritis and may be a manifestation of this disease.

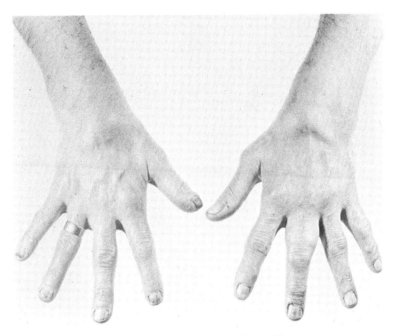

Figure 14 Synovial swelling of rheumatoid arthritis affecting extra-articular tissues; the extensor sheath of the right middle finger and the extensor communis sheaths on the backs of the wrists.

PRACTICAL POINTS

- Always look at the hands before any other physical examination.
- The 'rheumatic hand' is a part of many generalized conditions such as osteoarthrosis, rheumatoid arthritis, gout, neurological disorders and scleroderma.
- The hand may also reflect the personality of the patient, and/or some medical disorder other than arthritis, for instance:
  —A fine tremor may be a sign of senility, or nervousness, of Parkinsonism, of hyperthyroidism, or of alcoholic excess
  —A moist pink palm is common in rheumatoid arthritis but is also known as a 'liver' palm in chronic liver disease; it also occurs in normal but perhaps somewhat nervous subjects
  —Bitten finger nails and fingers heavily stained by cigarette smoking suggest nervous tension and 'fidgetiness'
  —The finger nail may show clubbing, pitting, ridging, discoloration or small haemorrhages suggesting other disorders ranging from lung disease to psoriasis, vasculitis or to bacterial endocarditis
  —The palmar contraction of Dupuytren is obvious, but a similar contraction may take place with rheumatoid arthritis.

4

The painful hip

A joint must allow movement between the bones that it unites while maintaining the stability of their union in the face of stress. Upper limb joints tend to favour mobility at the expense of stability. Lower limb joints which have to support the weight of the body tend to favour stability rather than mobility. The shoulder has a much wider range of movement than the hip but is much more easily dislocated.

The hip is mainly a supporter with the head of the femur locked into the solid bone of the pelvis and retained there by strong ligaments with the help of powerful muscles. Its mobility is necessarily limited and such movements as it has are easily compromised by underuse or misuse. The effect of underuse may be so insidious that many older people in our Western society are unaware that they have any disability even though the only hip movement that remains to them is flexion to a right angle. A disability of this kind would be obvious but unusual among people who are accustomed to the Buddha position of sitting on the ground with both hips externally rotated rather than spending most of their days seated on chairs, with hips flexed at right angles.

INFLAMMATORY DISEASES IN THE HIP

The hip joint may be affected by many types of inflammatory disease including rheumatoid, psoriatic, septic and tuberculous arthritis, and ankylosing spondylitis, but the degenerative changes which we describe as 'secondary osteoarthrosis' are by far the commonest cause of hip disability in developed countries. They may follow congenital dislocations, slipped epiphyses, badly set fractures, caisson disease, sickle cell anaemia and such hereditary disorders as ochronosis. This list is by no means exhaustive but with increasing knowledge of the conditions which may lead to osteoarthrosis there is a progressive diminution in the number of cases which we are constrained to describe as 'primary' or 'idiopathic'. Osteoarthrosis of the hip usually gets worse gradually. It may be unilateral at first but the second hip often follows the same course.

The possibility of an endocrine or a metabolic underlying disorder must always be considered.

Clinical features

Pain   Pain may be felt over the anterior aspect of the hip but there is a tendency for

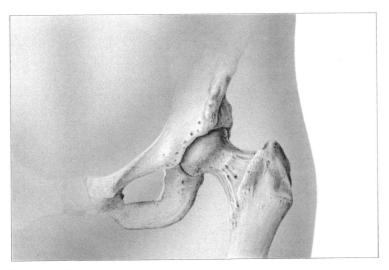

Figure 15 The anatomy of the hip.

pain to 'throw downward' in this area: disease of the sacro-iliac or lumbar spinal joints may cause pain in the hip, while disease of the hip may give rise to pain in the thigh or knee.

Pain may be aggravated by standing or walking, especially on a hard surface. It is increased when the sensitive capsule is stretched by full external or internal rotation. If there is acute synovitis with effusion, the position of greatest ease is with the hip flexed in slight external rotation. This fact presents a particular danger in children who adopt the position to avoid pain and may develop contractures within a few weeks. A sagging bed and mattress may allow this to occur without the patient or the doctor realizing what is happening.

The pain of osteoarthrosis is less severe in middle-aged or older patients who restrict their mobility to avoid it and tend to walk with the foot everted.

Stiffness limits the range of movements, especially those of rotation, abduction and adduction. Limitation of flexion and extension is less obvious but can be detected on examination. The gradual stiffening which commonly occurs in osteoarthrosis is hardly noticed by the patient who modifies his activities almost subconsciously and may be surprised to find that he is no longer able to perform movements that he once took for granted.

Weakness   The quadriceps wastes quickly, even in osteoarthrosis, and the former athlete may resent the feebleness of his thighs. Gait is affected, the body lurching towards the affected side. A combination of weakness, pain and contracture force the sufferer to a variety of complicated movements when he tries to sit down in a low chair

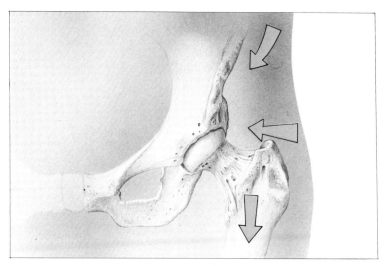

Figure 16   Pain sites at the hip – pain tending to be referred downwards from the lower lumbar spine to the hip and from the hip to the thigh and knee.

or to rise from it, to climb on to a bed or get in and out of a car, but he will experience his worst problems with an arthritic hip in the bathroom, where structural modifications and complicated manoeuvres can only postpone the day when the bath must be replaced by a shower.

Diagnosis

Diagnosis may be confused by the following:

1. **Disease of the sacro-iliac or lumbar spinal joints.**
2. **Acute inflammation of a trochanteric or iliopectineal bursa.** The pain of trochanteric bursitis is localized to the outer side of the hip and causes pain when the patient lies on that side. Pain is aggravated by abduction and by descending or ascending stairs. The iliopectineal bursa lies between the iliopsoas and the inguinal ligament. When it is inflamed the patient complains of pain radiating from the groin to the knee. He may walk with short strides to avoid overextension of the hip and tenderness may be found immediately below the inguinal ligament.
3. **Bone disorders,** especially Paget's disease and malignant deposits, whether primary or secondary.
4. **Inguinal hernia or lymphadenitis.**

Treatment

Treatment of the painful arthritic hip is directed at the underlying condition. It should include exercises, physiotherapy, walking aids and sticks, modification of furniture at home and work, alteration of automobile seats and appropriate use of analgesics and NSAIDs (see relevant chapters in Part 5).

Bursitis in the region of the hip is quite common in rheumatoid arthritis and may be treated by corticosteroid injection.

Surgery   Whether the cause of the patient's disability is osteoarthrosis, rheumatoid arthritis, ankylosing spondylitis or some other arthopathy, the time may come when surgical treatment has to be recommended. If the patient's general health permits, hip replacement should be considered whenever the pain and disability have become so great that life is a burden. There is a 5–10 per cent chance of an unsatisfactory result and a 1–2 per cent chance of thrombo-embolic disaster.

PRACTICAL POINTS

- Hip disease may be an isolated monarthrosis or part of a general arthropathic condition, inflammatory or degenerative.
- Symptoms are often referred to the hip from the sacro-iliac or lumbar spinal joints or from the hip to the thigh or knee.
- Clinical and radiological examination will usually lead to a correct diagnosis if the possibility of a soft tissue lesion is not forgotten.
- A patient with osteoarthrosis of the hip is likely to benefit from NSAIDs given in adequate doses but may be helped to at least an equal extent by advice about modification of his environment and the use of special aids.
- The operation of hip replacement can relieve many patients, whether their disease is degenerative or inflammatory and whether or not other joints are affected. The correct time for it is probably 'as late as possible'.

5
The knee

The knees are the joints most often involved in injuries and rheumatic disorders. Built as they are chiefly for walking and running involving flexion and extension, they are also subjected to twisting and lateral strains causing injury. They are weight-bearing joints and so obesity may cause strain. Also, the knees are involved early in generalized joint disorders and systemic diseases.

There is much more to knee disorders than trauma, osteoarthrosis and rheumatoid disease. A whole number of other conditions may cause pain, swelling and loss of function.

APPLIED ANATOMY AND PATHOLOGY

The mobility of the knee joint is limited by the need for stability when bearing weight. Its range of movement is confined to flexion and extension with a slight forward sliding of the femur on the tibia when walking.

The joint has medial and lateral, anterior and posterior compartments, the femur articulating with the patella in front and the tibia below (see diagram opposite). It is surrounded by bursae; the semimembranosus (popliteal), the semitendinosus and the supra-, pre- and infrapatellar bursae. Of these the semimembranosus communicates with the joint through a valve-like opening which allows fluid to enter the bursa but not to return. It is an overflow tank for the knee. The suprapatellar bursa also communicates with the joint.

The patella is a large sesamoid bone with sensitive tendinous and ligamentous attachments. It may be fractured or dislocated. The fibula is attached to the tibia by a synarthrodial joint, which is important for stability and normal function. The medial and lateral menisci are cartilaginous cushions between the femur and tibia. If they are torn, and particularly if portions come to lie loose in the joint, they are likely to cause locking of the knee and may have to be removed. This is a common athletic injury, especially in footballers.

As the owner of the knee ages, the cartilage at the back of the patella ages with him, and the degree of patellofemoral change corresponds roughly with the age of the

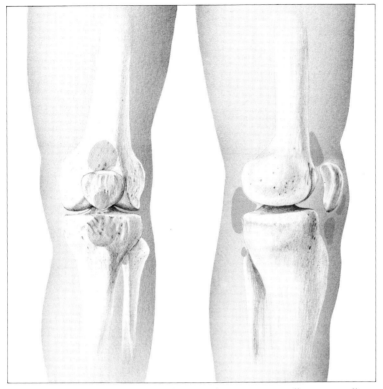

Figure 17 Knee compartments: the main bursae – supratellar, prepatellar, infrapatellar, semimembranosus (Baker's cyst), bursa of the popliteal tendon.

patient, unless there are abnormal stresses, strains or postural defects. Bow legs or knock-knees, for instance, may date from early life, whether they are due to congenital defect, injury or vitamin deficiency. Obesity imposes additional strain, not only from increased weight but also from postural defects when fat thighs and pendulous abdomen throw extra strain on the knees both in standing and in walking.

The essential pathological changes of the more common disorders (osteoarthrosis and rheumatoid arthritis) involve the bones, cartilaginous covering and the synovial lining of the joint (Figures 18 and 19).

In osteoarthrosis the characteristic changes are atrophic thinning and wear of the cartilage, sclerosis of the underlying bone and osteophytic hypertrophy and roughening of the tibia and femur.

In rheumatoid arthritis the main early changes are in the synovium with inflammatory cell infiltration and swelling. This pannus spreads across the cartilage eroding and eventually destroying it.

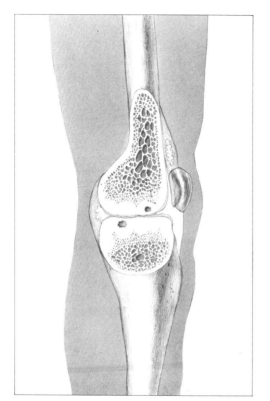

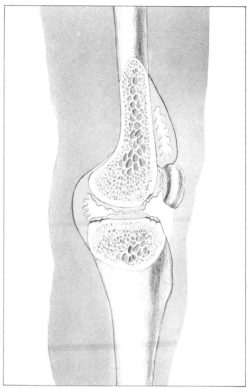

Figure 18 The knee is osteoarthrosis: there is eburnation of the bone beneath the degenerated cartilage. Synovial proliferation is much less than in rheumatoid arthritis and here is demonstrated by moderate proliferation posteriorly and in the suprapatellar pouch. Small bone cysts (geodes) may be present close to the joint.

Figure 19 Rheumatoid knee shown here in an early inflamed stage with synovial and bursal proliferation, particularly of the suprapatellar bursa, and early erosive changes in bone and cartilage.

EXAMINATION OF THE KNEE: SOME HELPFUL SIGNS

Crepitus behind the patella in the patellofemoral compartment. This can be felt and often heard (best with a stethoscope). In middle age or later it is usually due to osteoarthrosis and is of small significance, but in the young it may be due to chondromalacia patellae (see page 39). If the examiner holds the patella distally without pressing it on to the femur and then asks the patient to contract his quadriceps there should be a strong, painless contraction against resistance. A poor contraction accompanied by discomfort suggests disease.

Fluid in a knee may be seen as a bulging which can be compressed from one area to another either by pressing on the lateral side to produce a visible bulge medially or by ballottement between the examiner's hands above and below the patella, squeezing fluid from hand to hand. Patellar tapping in which the floating patella is tapped back against the femur is found in the presence of fluid but occurs in some normal joints.

Points of tenderness may be found after injury. The line of the cartilage on the medial side is often tender in osteo- or rheumatoid arthritis. The tibial tubercle may be tender in Osgood-Schlatter disease (osteochondritis) – in adolescent boys more often than girls.

Posterior swelling may be found on one or both sides, the semimembranosus bursa enlarging by overflow from a joint effusion. If this Baker's cyst or popliteal bursa ruptures, fluid may extravasate into the calf. In rheumatoid arthritis this produces a low-grade inflammation which is easily mistaken for thrombophlebitis. The diagnosis may be difficult because popliteal phlebothrombosis may be associated with large knee effusions.

Instability of the knee may be the result of injury or inflammation. Lateral instability is quite common in rheumatoid arthritis. Anterior instability is due to an incompetent anterior cruciate ligament and posterior instability to posterior cruciate deficiency. The former is much more common.

Quadriceps strength and tone can be checked by palpating the muscle when contracted and relaxed and by testing movement against resistance. The girth of the thigh should be compared with that of the opposite limb by measuring at similar levels above the upper border of the patella.

Temperature can be estimated by hand in the usual way. A joint inflamed by rheumatoid arthritis or by trauma may be warm. Greater heat suggests a more acute inflammation such as pyarthrosis or gout.

The standing and walking patient may show defects of stance and gait, genu valgum varum or recurvatum, and perhaps leg shortening. The shoes may show uneven wear (see Chapter 6).

Aspirate synovial fluid if still in doubt, in order to check cell count, viscosity, micro-organisms and possibly crystals. Normal joint fluid has up to 50 white cells per cu mm but counts of up to 2,000 may be found in conditions such as osteoarthrosis, which do give rise to low-grade inflammatory episodes, even though they are essentially degenerative. Inflammatory fluids, as in rheumatoid arthritis, are less viscous than normal and contain more than 2,000 cells per cu mm. Counts over 60,000 suggest bacterial infection although counts up to 100,000 do occur in some cases of Reiter's disease, and rheumatoid or crystal-induced arthritis. Polymorphs are fewer than 25 per cent of the total cells in normal subjects and in noninflammatory conditions, over 50 per cent in inflammatory conditions and over 75 per cent in the case of septic infections.

THE SWOLLEN PAINFUL KNEE

Background

A very common problem presentation in practice is that of a painful and swollen knee.

The following collection of clinical possibilities is divided into common (at least once a year), rare (once every five to ten years), and very rare (once or twice in one's professional lifetime in general practice).

Common
- Trauma
- Chondromalacia patellae
- Osteoarthrosis
- Rheumatoid arthritis
- Pre- or infrapatellar bursitis
- Nonarthritis

Uncommon
- Gout or pseudogout
- Osteochondritis dissecans
- Intermittent hydrarthrosis
- Pyarthrosis
- Synovial chondromatosis
- Pseudohypertrophic pulmonary osteoarthropathy
- Reiter's disease
- Bleeding states (haemophilia, etc)

Very uncommon
- Clutton's joints
- Neuropathic (Charcot's) joints
- Malignant disease
- Synovial haemangiomas
- Scurvy
- Sarcoidosis
- Pigmental villonodular synovitis
- Fatty synovial lesions (Hoffa's disease)

Common syndromes

Trauma The history will probably give the answer. A true haemarthrosis develops within minutes, while effusion takes hours.

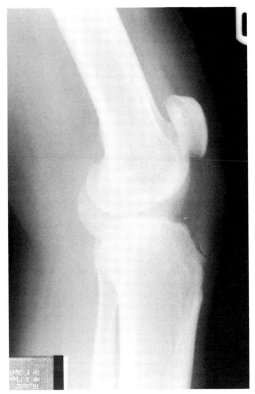

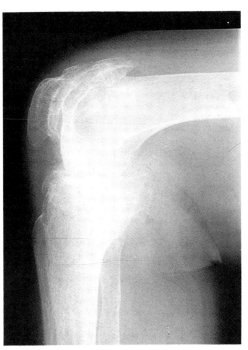

Figure 20 Erosive rheumatoid changes in the articular surface of the lower half of the patella in a man aged fifty, in contrast to the changes in younger subjects with chondromalacia patellae.

Figure 21 Lateral views of gross osteoarthrosis of the knees with marked osteophytosis.

Chondromalacia patellae may be a separate entity or may be a precursor of osteoarthrosis. The early lesion is in the midpart of the patella – between the lateral and medial facets – in the places where the patella is in contact with the femur during midflexion. It occurs early in life and may follow injury or be associated with unduly mobile patellae. Chondromalacia and recurrent subluxation often occur in the same patient who complains of pain behind the patella with recurrent swelling of the knee. There is pain on pressing over the patella and contracting the quadriceps.

Osteoarthrosis may occur in early life if there is congenital or acquired abnormality, but symptoms usually appear in middle life or later. The condition is more common in women and is associated with overweight.

The complaints are pain and stiffness, particularly after prolonged walking, standing or squatting. Descending stairs is usually more painful than ascending them. Pains may also occur after sitting and on moving the joints after immobility, particularly after

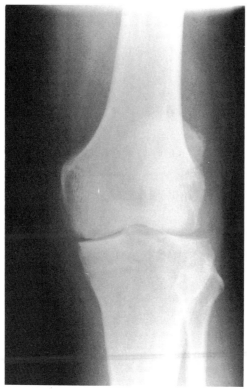

Figure 22   X-ray showing rheumatoid changes in the knee.

prolonged flexion. Pre-existent genu valgum or varum, possibly the result of rickets or poliomyelitis, may predispose to osteoarthrosis, but osteoarthrosis may itself be the cause of those deformities, usually valgum.

In osteoarthrosis the knees have a restricted range of flexion but are usually capable of full extension. Effusions may follow even mild trauma or be the result of deposition of calcium pyrophosphate or hydroxyapatite. Tenderness over the medial meniscus is common.

Rheumatoid arthritis of the knee may present with synovial proliferation, an effusion or both. As has been said, it is like palpating seaweed in sea water. Valgum deformity (knock-knee) is more common than varum (bow-leg). The joint may feel cold and clammy. The quadriceps is often weak and wasted. Bursae may be involved, particularly the semimembranosus at the back. Flexion and extension are often limited. Tenderness may be present, most often on the medial side, but it is seldom severe. There may be similar findings in seronegative arthritis, such as psoriatric arthropathy. Effusions may occur in ankylosing spondylitis, usually but not always early in its course.

Pre- or infrapatellar bursitis Also known as housemaid's knee, nun's, priest's or windowdresser's knee, this condition is due to prepatellar or infrapatellar bursitis from friction which is usually unrelated to arthritis. These and other bursae may be involved in any inflammatory polyarthritis, bursitis being part of the inflammatory polyarthritic process when the knee is affected. Prepatellar bursitis over the front of the knee lies between the patella and the skin and is easily traumatized by frequent kneeling. As with infrapatellar bursitis, it is unlikely to be confused with hydrarthrosis.

Nonarthritis Pain may be referred to the knee from the hip or spine when no disease is present in the knee itself. It is quite common for patients to complain of pain in the knee, which is normal, and not of the hip which is highly abnormal. Similarly, pains from a femoral neuropathy (as in diabetic amyotrophy) may be referred to knee and thigh.

Uncommon syndromes

Gout or pseudogout may cause acute painful inflammatory effusion in the knee due to deposition of monosodium urate or calcium pyrophosphate dihydrate (CPPD). Pseudogout due to CPPD may occur apparently primarily or secondary to some other disorder such as hyperparathyroidism or haemochromatosis. Both uratic gout and pseudogout may be precipitated by trauma, a surgical operation or an acute illness. The knee is a common site for CPPD deposition but an uncommon site for true gout. Diagnosis is confirmed by examination of aspirated fluid with a polarizing microscope. X-rays show calcification of cartilages in CPPD. In true gout there are usually no X-ray changes, but very rarely there are punched-out areas of uratic deposition. Diabetes often co-exists with pseudogout but seldom with true gout.

Osteochondritis dissecans is characterized by separation of avascular fragments of bone from articular surfaces. It can occur at any age but is most usual between ten and twenty years. Swelling may come and go, the knee feeling unstable, locking and giving way. X-rays show separation of fragments of bone from the joint surface, the commonest site being the lateral border of the medial condyle of the femur. Half these patients develop osteoarthrosis in later life.

Intermittent hydrarthrosis Effusions into the knee occur at intervals. In some cases the condition proves to be an early manifestation of rheumatoid arthritis, ankylosing spondylitis or Reiter's disease, but in others the effusions cease to occur, with no sign of arthritis in any joint. It differs from palindromic rheumatism in that it is usually confined to one knee and the attacks occur fairly regularly. Effusions may be quite large with fluid containing fewer than 6,000 cells per cu mm – predominantly mononuclears. Biopsy reveals only a nonspecific synovitis. Effusions usually last two to six days and recur every one to three weeks.

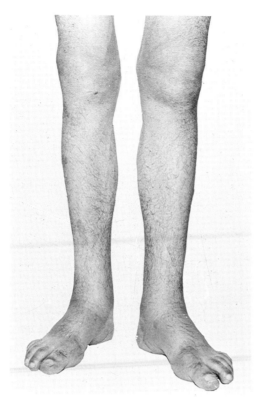

Figure 23 Knee effusions in a man suffering from pseudohypertrophic pulmonary osteoarthropathy due to a bronchial carcinoma.

Pyarthrosis The joint is painful, swollen, hot and red. Destructive changes may occur rapidly but the earliest X-ray changes are not seen for ten days or more. Aspiration and culture must be followed by treatment with the appropriate antibiotic, systemically and sometimes into the joint. Surgical drainage is often necessary. Pyarthrosis may complicate rheumatoid arthritis.

Synovial chondromatosis is a rare, benign, self-limiting disease affecting the young and middle-aged – usually males – in which the joint space fills up with free-floating cartilaginous bodies. The knee is the joint most frequently involved. Features are pain, swelling, stiffness and crepitus. X-rays show free-floating opacities associated with synovial thickening or intrasynovial soft tissue masses, but in some cases calcification is not seen because not all the cartilaginous bodies calcify or ossify. Treatment is by surgical excision.

Pseudohypertophic pulmonary osteoarthropathy may affect the knee which is swollen with effusion but not very painful. Clubbing of the fingers is usually present and there is often swelling of the ankles. This condition is nearly always a manifestation of malignant disease elsewhere, commonly a subpleural (peripheral) carcinoma of bronchus. No malignant process is present in the joints, whose condition improves rapidly if the neoplasm is removed. X-rays show new bone laid down under the periosteum in the forearms, and the legs below the knee. The diagnostic sign is clubbing of the fingers and sometimes the toes.

Reiter's disease is more common in males (20:1) and usually occurs between the ages of 18 and 40. Knees (90 per cent), ankles (75 per cent) and feet are involved more often than the upper limbs. Urethritis is or has been present in most cases but conjunctivitis is often transient or absent. A history of venereal exposure or dysentery ten to twelve days beforehand can usually be obtained by questioning.

Joint effusions may be present and the disease may be very acute and painful or subacute. It usually resolves within a few weeks but sometimes relapses. Occasionally it becomes chronic. There may be skin lesions on the penis and ulcers in the mouth. Skin lesions (keratodermia blennorrhagica) may be found on the lower extremities. They have a close resemblance to psoriasis, both clinically and histologically.

Bleeding states   Haemophilia and other haemorrhagic disorders may cause bleeding into the knees with acute pain and distension. The diagnosis is made by haematological examination and aspiration of the joint. Leukaemic involvement of the knee in children is usually misdiagnosed as Still's disease (see Chapter 11). Haemarthrosis may be caused by medicinal anticoagulants.

Very uncommon syndromes

Clutton's joints are now almost a thing of the past. There is hydrarthrosis of the knees associated with congenital syphilis and occurring at any age between six and eighteen years. This condition may be confused with Still's disease or with juvenile ankylosing spondylitis. The swelling is usually bilateral and asymmetrical. Serological tests for syphilis are positive.

Neuropathic (Charcot's) joints are now period pieces in developed countries. If occurring in the knee they may be due to syphilis (tabes dorsalis) or, less often, to leprosy or yaws. The diagnostic feature is freedom from severe pain in spite of the gross disorganization of the joint which results from repeated trauma. In syphilitic cases there are usually other signs of tabes and a positive serology. The patient is usually aged forty to seventy. Males predominate in a ratio of 3:2.

Malignant disease   Synovioma (synovial sarcoma) is a very rare, highly malignant growth which arises in the synovium, usually that of the knee. There is pain in 60 per

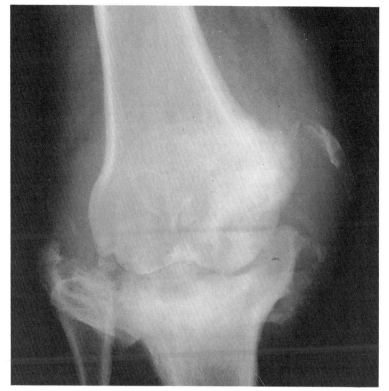

Figure 24   Charcot's neuropathic knee, secondary to tabes dorsalis.

cent of cases. Soft tissue and joint swelling come on insidiously at any age but usually between twenty and sixty years, with a mean age of thirty-two. Metastasis is common and prognosis bad with only 10 per cent of the patients alive after ten years. Other varities of sarcoma also occur, eg, liposarcoma and Paget sarcoma of bone. Metastases from other parts of the body are very rarely deposited in the knee.

Synovial haemangioma is a very rare benign tumour of joints in children and young adults. The knee is affected in 95 per cent of cases. If the tumour is localized there are episodes of pain in the joint which locks or gives way from time to time and the swelling is localized, appearing and disappearing at intervals. Synovial fluid is blood-stained. If the tumour is diffuse the joint is diffusely swollen and there may be episodes of pain associated with haemarthrosis. The swollen knee feels doughy and compressible, and its bulk may diminish when the limb is elevated. There may be a haemangioma of the overlying skin.

Scurvy is rare but it may cause pain and swelling of joints, most commonly the knees and hips. Pain may be intense in infants who scream when their joints are moved. In adults there is usually swelling and dull aching. Haemorrhages in the mouth and under the skin are common. Nowadays scorbutic patients are often on a special restricted diet or are chronic alcoholics or food faddists.

Sarcoidosis may cause pain and swelling in several joints, but knees and ankles are the most commonly affected. Erythema nodosum is frequently associated with sarcoidosis and X-ray of the chest shows bilateral hilar adenopathy (see Figure 58).

Pigmented villonodular synovitis is a very rare nonmalignant condition characterized by marked synovial proliferation, pigmentation with haemosiderin and the formation of nodular, grape-like masses. This condition is essentially a chronic synovitis of only one knee joint but it may involve bursae and tendon sheath and even capsule and bone. Although behaving almost like a neoplasm it never metastasizes. The aetiology is unknown. Repeated episodes of dark bloody effusion are very suggestive of this condition, which usually affects young adults.

Fatty synovial lesions   In this condition, also called Hoffa's disease, and lipoarthritis traumatica genu, pain seems to arise from the fringe of the infrapatellar pad of fat becoming swollen and incarcerated in the joint. It is said to occur in ballet dancers and acrobats, usually after an injury, and to be relieved by excision of the fatty pad. On examination there is tenderness below the patella but the knee is otherwise normal.

A true lipoma of the joint is rare. More common is the lipoma arborescens, a benign lipomatous mass that occurs most commonly in the knee. It is usually associated with degenerative changes and occurs most frequently in the suprapatellar or lateral pouch. It may cause pain, locking and restricted movement with effusion. If there is swelling it becomes more evident on full flexion of the knee. Surgical removal may be necessary.

What to do

1. General principles   Before even considering the nature and type of knee disorder it is necessary to consider the patient's normal occupation and the extent to which the disorder is interfering with normal activities, and how strains on the knees may be relieved.

General commonsense matters must include attention to overweight, exercise and muscle building of quadriceps, hobbies and recreational activities.

2. Management of effusion   Treatment of the painful swollen knee will depend on the disorder affecting it, but the big decision will be whether to encourage or restrain activity. If an acute effusion is greatly affecting function, is unpleasantly painful or is holding up progress in osteoarthrosis or an inflammatory arthropathy, aspiration followed by injection of a long-acting corticosteroid is usually helpful (see Chapters 30 and 31).

3. Use of drugs The use of analgesics or nonsteroidal anti-inflammatory drugs (NSAIDs) will depend on the diagnosis and the requirements of individual patients, but if a joint is acutely painful and inflamed, rest is essential – with analgesics, NSAIDs or both being given as indicated. An inflammatory arthropathy will probably need regular NSAIDs with simple analgesics added as required to cover painful episodes. Osteo-arthrosis can usually be treated with analgesics as required, only adding an NSAID if pain is severe during much of the day rather than being occasional and episodic. Some patients, however, derive more relief from NSAIDs than from simple analgesics, even though their pain is episodic (see Chapter 29).

4. Exercise and activity must be suited to the individual patient, but if no acute inflammation is present at least some degree of mobility and regular exercise is desirable in either osteoarthrosis or rheumatoid arthritis (see Chapter 32). Together with weight reduction, it is particularly necessary for fat, lethargic, elderly osteo-arthrotics.

5. Physiotherapy, at home or in the clinic, will help to maintain function and morale, but like any other treatment, including medication, it should not be continued for long periods unless some benefit is seen to arise from it. The timing of any form of therapy in relation to patient and disease activity is as crucial to success as the actual treatment given.

6. Surgery Surgical procedures may be helpful in some of the conditions such as removal of damaged menisci, possible replacement of the joint or arthrodesis in severe osteoarthrosis or rheumatoid disease, synovectomy in rheumatoid disease, osteotomy in osteoarthrosis with deformity and removal of loose bodies in osteochondritis dissecans or chondromatosis.

However, in most conditions surgery plays a small part.

7. Home care In any chronic arthritis the home management of the case must include:

1. Instruction as to what and how much exercise, exercises and periods of rest should be taken. Some patients need encouragement to maintain or extend their mobility. Only a minority have to be restrained from doing too much.
2. Instruction in home physiotherapy, heat and exercises, and use of local rubs, counterirritants and rubefacient creams.
3. Modification of home and working conditions, with adaptation of furniture and use of helpful gadgets.
4. Instruction about the medicines to be taken.
5. Advice about the social services available.

PRACTICAL POINTS

- Knees are prone to trauma and disease. Pain and swelling may be from a local discrete disorder or they may be part of a more general systemic disease.
- Effects of knee disorders may cause much disability and loss of function because they are so important in locomotion.
- Definition of the cause of the problem may be helped by examination of synovial fluid aspirate.
- The most common knee disorders are:
  —Trauma
  —Osteoarthrosis and chondromalacia patellae
  —Rheumatoid arthritis
  —Bursitis
- Many of the less common disorders are part of general systemic disorders.
- Management should include:
  —**Noting** personal and family problems and situation; nature of occupation and leisure activities; weight; and general health
  —**Aspiration** of effusion and injection of corticosteroids into the joint often produce rapid relief of pain
  —**Drugs**: analgesics and NSAIDs often used
  —**Exercise**: relate to individual and the condition
  —**Physiotherapy**: may help but is not a panacea
  —**Surgery**: may help in a few instances.

6
The foot

The feet bear much weight in the human animal. Even minor disorders can cause major function disturbance. It is important, therefore, to be able to diagnose and manage foot problems.

Feet are born flat and develop towards the adult form as a child grows. As with the hand, function is more important than shape or appearance but a spot diagnosis can often be made as soon as the shoes and socks have been removed. One sock can hide a dozen important medical conditions, some of which are arthritic.

THE CONDITIONS

The osteoarthrotic foot

This is very common in white women but may occur in males and in people with darker skins. The osteoarthrosis is usually due to deformity caused by bad shoes. Advice is most often sought because of hallux valgus with an overlying bunion on one foot or both.

The rheumatoid foot

A normal foot will withstand badly fitting shoes for years, but a foot affected by rheumatoid arthritis – where muscles are weakened, ligaments are lax and cartilages and bones are eroded – may become deformed in weeks or months. Hallux valgus leads to crushing of the smaller toes so that one or more of their proximal interphalangeal joints scrape on the underside of the toe-caps of the shoes and become hardened or eroded, while the tips of the terminal phalanges press down on the sole. Figure 27

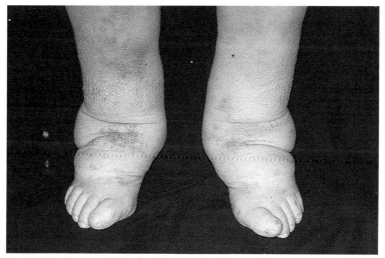

Figure 25   Osteoarthrotic feet in a grossly obese subject.

shows the three abnormal pressure points: on the head of the metatarsal, on the proximal interphalangeal joints and on the tip of the toe.

The longitudinal and transverse arches tend to flatten with the forefoot moving laterally on midtarsus, the foot everting and the medial malleolus dropping (see Figures 28 and 29). The general effect is for the rheumatoid patient to walk flatly and painfully with the 'Charlie Chaplin' gait of First World War infantrymen. Deforming rheumatoid disease in ankle, knee and hip add postural strain to the foot and increase the patient's misery. Vascular, nodular and neuropathic changes bring further hazards, sometimes with erosion or even gangrene. Callosities and painful areas are common at hardened pressure points.

Rheumatoid arthritis may affect the ankle and the midtarsal, tarsometatarsal and metatarsophalangeal joints. The interphalangeal joints are seldom affected by rheumatoid arthritis but they are damaged by posture and positional changes. The small bursae between the heads of the second, third, fourth and fifth metatarsals become inflamed and exert pressure on adjacent bone and soft tissues. Even when the metatarsal heads are only slightly tender to pressure, compressing the foot between finger and thumb is usually uncomfortable or actually painful. The tendo Achillis may be affected at its insertion into the os calcis with tenderness and sometimes with painful nodules. Inspection of the shoes will give further information about the foot because bulgings and irregular wear deform the shoes.

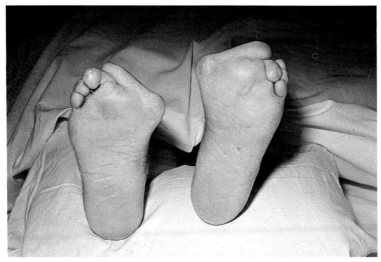

Figure 26 Feet in rheumatoid arthritis showing typical distortion of toes laterally, prominent metatarsal heads and fallen arches with area of skin thickening at the base of the third right metatarsal.

Figure 27 Three abnormal pressure points in deformed foot.

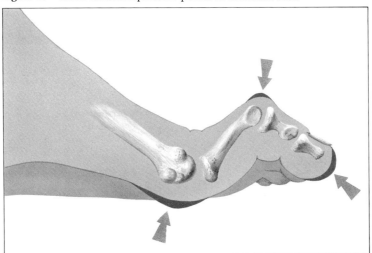

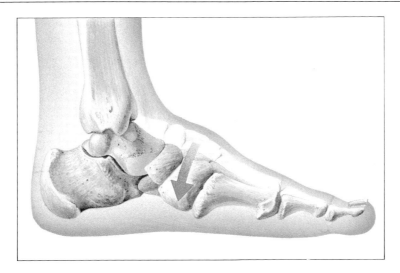

Figure 28   Fallen arch in flat foot.

Figure 29   Foot everting and medial malleolus dropping in rheumatoid flat foot.

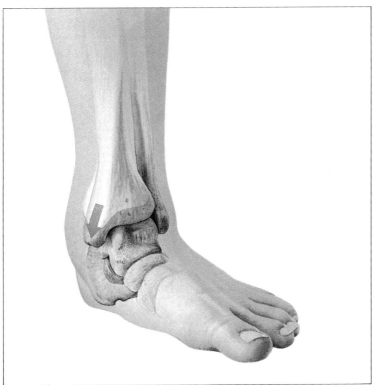

The gouty foot

Acute gout occurs most commonly in the metatarsophalangeal joint of the big toe. The part is swollen, tender, red and shining. The pain is agonizing. As the inflammation subsides after two to seven days the superficial layers of the skin often flake off. Similar changes may occur in the midtarsus or ankle. The chronic tophaceous gouty foot is now rarely seen. The illustrations opposite show the foot of a man who had three attacks of gout in the feet and then, at the age of sixty-one, developed tophi in the areas affected. There is bulging and thickening of the tissues with typical tophaceous material showing through the skin in places.

The seronegative arthritic foot

In Reiter's disease the feet and ankles may become so painfully inflamed that gout is suspected. Tenderness of the os calcis is common, at the insertion of the tendo Achillis and/or that of the plantar fascia. These sites may also be affected in ankylosing spondylitis but the manifestations are usually episodic and do not last for long. The interphalangeal joints, seldom involved in rheumatoid arthritis, are often affected in Reiter's disease and psoriatic arthropathy, giving the sausage-shaped inflamed toe. The skin rashes in psoriasis and Reiter's disease are similar to one another, both clinically and histologically. Toe-nails may show yellow colouring and coarse ridging in both diseases.

The young athletic foot

This may suffer from interdigital fungus infection. Sweating may be aggravated by tight, synthetic-fibre socks, by plastic or rubber shoes, or by foam-plastic linings. Unsuitable footwear may produce friction areas, callosities and corns.

The neglected foot of old age

This may suffer from osteoarthrosis and also from deformed toe-nails (onychogryphosis), untended pressure points, infection beneath ingrowing nails, skin infection between the toes and poor arterial supply. Socks and shoes that once fitted may no longer do so. The transverse arch may flatten out and the protective pads under the metatarsophalangeals may atrophy. The elderly and osteoarthritic are often unable to reach their own feet to care for them and if help is not available the feet suffer and the whole patient suffers with them.

The neuropathic foot

The neuropathic foot with diminished or absent sensory functions arises most commonly in diabetics or alcoholics but may occur with any peripheral neuritis. Such changes are rarely found in rheumatoid arthritis, systemic lupus erythematosus and polyarteritis nodosa. Diabetes and alcoholism are so common that they frequently coexist with other disorders.

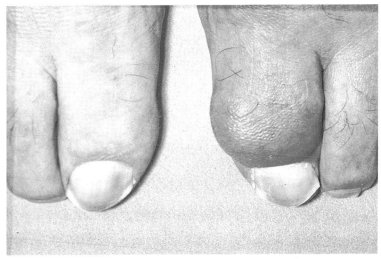

Figure 30   Acute gout in the left big toe.

Figure 31   Tophaceous gout over heel and base of little toe.

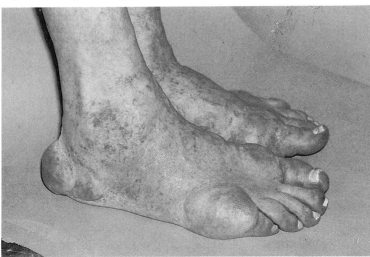

The injured foot

After a fracture, sprain or minor injury the cause of local pain, tenderness and swelling is usually obvious. March fractures may have to be sought by radiography. The second metatarsal is their usual but not only site.

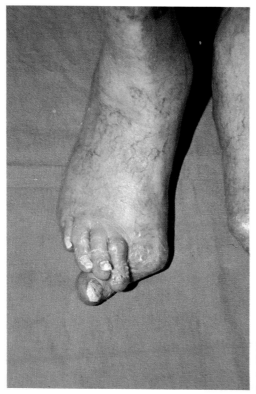

Figure 32 A neglected foot with gross hallux valgus. Many elderly patients cannot properly care for their own feet as they cannot reach them.

PRACTICAL POINTS

● In rheumatoid arthritis the feet are often affected and cause serious functional problems.
● In old age the feet may be affected through neglect and inability to care for them.
● The neuropathic foot in diabetes and in alcoholics may lead to ulceration, infection and gangrene.

7
Young backache

Backache predominates in adults – particularly in middle age. Backache in children is unusual and if persistent must be taken seriously.

In childhood and adolescence the more likely causes are congenital abnormalities and injuries. Infections such as tuberculosis, osteomyelitis or subdural and epidural infections are now rare. Note rare but possible neoplastic lesions.

Young children (under ten)

Children in this age group rarely complain of backache and when they do there must be a strong suspicion of local organic disease.

Infection may spread from a vertebral body to cause 'discitis' with a narrowed intervertebral space on X-ray.

Osteoid osteoma is another rarity that is more often found in the femur and tibia than in the spine. It is a minute benign tumour which may cause anything from mild to severe pain, often worse at night but eased by aspirin. Although said to be most common in adolescent boys it may occur at earlier or later ages. X-rays show a radiolucent core, sharply demarcated from a zone of sclerotic bone which surrounds it. The core itself may become calcified. Removal of this small lesion effects a cure.

Older children (ten to fifteen)

In older children, as in adults, backache may be the result of mental stress or be a deliberate or half-conscious ploy to escape from an awkward situation such as having to go to school, play games or sit an exam. Organic conditions do, however, occur, and the following are the more frequent ones.

ORGANIC SPINAL CONDITIONS IN OLDER CHILDREN

Spinal osteochondritis

Also known as Scheuermann's disease, this condition may affect adolescent males. It is a condition of unknown aetiology in which there is irregular ossification of the vertebral epiphyseal end-plates in the lower dorsal and, to a lesser extent, the upper lumbar spine. The youth often has an ache in this area and it tends to increase as he ages and secondary changes occur. He has dorsal kyphosis, round shoulders and a flat chest. X-rays are characteristic:

1. The disc spaces are narrowed in the lower dorsal spine and the vertebral bodies become wedged anteriorly.
2. There is fragmentation of the epiphyseal plates with increased density and irregularity of the edge of the vertebral bodies.
3. Multiple herniations of the nuclei pulposi into the vertebral bodies often occur through these weakened areas (Schmorl's nodes).

In some cases the patient should wear a well-fitting brace until the time when skeletal maturity is reached but the majority need no more than symptomatic treatment.

Juvenile chronic polyarthritis (Still's disease)

This does not often cause backache, although the neck and hips may be severely involved, becoming very stiff and painful (see also Chapter 11). Although this disease is still called 'rheumatoid juvenile polyarthritis' in some parts of the world, Dr Barbara Ansell's[1] careful follow up of children whom she and Prof Bywaters had observed for many years has shown that most of these children remain seronegative for rheumatoid factor and that only about 8 per cent grow on to adult rheumatoid arthritis. Around 10 per cent, however, most of them boys, develop ankylosing spondylitis in their teens.

Ankylosing spondylitis

If this starts in early adult life its main symptom is backache and pain in the buttocks with spinal stiffness; but if the disease begins between the ages of nine and fourteen the chief complaint is usually not of backache but of pains and effusions in the knees and other joints of the lower extremities, the classical adult symptoms only occurring later when sacro-iliac joint changes appear in X-rays, usually between the ages of eighteen and twenty-two.

Juvenile ankylosing spondylitis

This condition is six times as common in boys as in girls but when it does occur in girls the symptoms are similar. In my own experience hydrarthrosis of the knees, and pain and swelling of the ankles and feet are common early manifestations. Two boys, aged

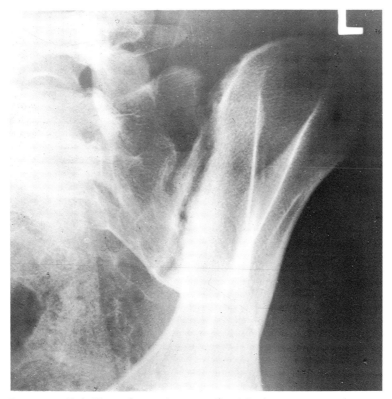

Figure 33   Early X-ray changes in a sacro-iliac joint in a young man;
taken in an oblique position to show early erosive changes and partial
fusion of the lower third with 'eagle's wing' changes in the upper third,
calcification beginning to appear in the ligamentous attachments.

twelve and thirteen had acute swelling of the big toe, reminiscent of adult gout.

In Ansell's series around 10 per cent of children with 'juvenile chronic polyarthritis' developed ankylosing spondylitis. Only five had backache and in only one was this the first complaint. Hips were commonly involved early. Joints of the upper limb were seldom affected, hands and wrists in only 8 per cent. A family history of ankylosing spondylitis or acute iridocyclitis was quite common, being elicited from a third of families on direct questioning. Ninety per cent of these patients were HLA$_{B27}$ positive. By the time the child has become a young adult the pattern of symptoms and radiological changes has usually made the diagnosis obvious.

Scoliosis

This condition is not uncommon in childhood. A lateral deviation of the spine may be nonstructural, disappearing on flexing the spine, or structural and constant. Although the latter may cause backache later in life in young people, scoliosis is not accompanied by backache in most cases – though in some severe cases it is.

If it is reversible and not severe it is best left alone. But if it is irreversible, progressive and over 55–60°, reducing pulmonary efficiency, it may be treated by surgical fusion of the spine.

Spondylolysis and spondylolisthesis

In these conditions there is a break in bony continuity in the pars interarticularis in the posterior part of the child's spine, between superior and inferior facet joints (spondylolysis) which may lead to a slipping forward of one vertebral body on the one below (spondylolisthesis). This occurs most commonly between L5 and S1, sometimes between L4 and 5, rarely at higher levels. The condition may be congenital, acquired or both. It may be symptomless but there is often low back pain and this may worsen at periods of rapid growth causing root irritation at L5/S1, with impaired straight leg raising and spasm in the spinal and hamstring muscles. Spondylolysis may cause pain, especially in vigorous, athletic children aged ten to twelve, but spondylolisthesis is usually also present.

Lateral X-rays show a typical picture. Serial X-rays may reveal a progressive worsening, with forward slipping of displaced vertebrae. Spinal fusion then becomes necessary. Otherwise, treatment is by exercises to reduce lumbar lordosis and so reduce pain, avoidance of exertion associated with lumbar spinal extension, and support by a brace.

Other conditions

Reiter's disease, inflammatory bowel disease (Crohn's disease and ulcerative colitis) and psoriatic arthritis may all occur in childhood and early adult life, and in a minority of cases progress to the clinical picture of ankylosing spondylitis. Such patients are often HLAB_{27} positive (see also Chapter 8).

COMMON SPINAL CONDITIONS IN YOUNG ADULTS

Back strain, postural fatigue and injury account for most backaches between the ages of twenty and thirty but disc prolapses, which are more common at a later age, may occur in the twenties.

Back pain may then be due to stimulation of nerve roots or of sensory endings in the spine itself (see list of pain origin sites, opposite). The pathways from spinal receptors usually arise from several segments, causing the pain to be poorly localized and to

Sites of origin of spinal pain[2]

1. Skin and subcutaneous tissues.
2. Apophyseal and sacro-iliac joint capsules.
3. Longitudinal spinal ligaments, particularly the posterior longitudinal one.
4. Periosteum and attached fasciae, tendons and aponeuroses.
5. The dura mater and epidural adipose tissues.
6. The walls of blood vessels in and around the spine.

spread over a large area. The intervertebral disc has no sensory nerve endings but pain receptors are present around it in the outer edge of the annulus fibrosus particularly where it is attached to the posterior longitudinal ligament. The Table below gives a rough scheme of the neurological findings in disc prolapse at various levels.

Neurological signs of lumbar disc lesions

Root	Pain reference	Motor weakness	Sensory changes	Reflex change	Muscle wasting
L2	Anterior upper thigh	Flexion and adduction of hip	None or upper thigh (lateral and anterior)	None or reduced knee reflex	None
L3	Anterior thigh and knee	Knee extension, hip flexion and adduction	None or lower thigh (medial and anterior)	Reduced knee reflex	Thigh
L4	Lateral thigh, median calf	Foot inversion and dorsiflexion, knee extension	Anteromedial calf and shin	Reduced or absent knee reflex	Thigh
L5	Buttock, back and side thigh, lateral lower leg	Extension and abduction hip, flexion knee, dorsiflexion foot and toes, foot eversion	Lateral calf, dorsal and medial foot, especially hallux	Nil, or (rarely) reduced ankle reflex	Calf
S1	Buttock, back of thigh and calf to heel	Flexion knee foot eversion and plantar flexion	Lateral foot, ankle and lower calf, back of heel and sole of foot	Reduced or absent ankle reflex	Calf

PRACTICAL POINTS

● Backache is rare in young children without local organic disease. 'Discitis' or osteoid osteoma may be the cause.
● In teenagers remember as causes
  —Prolapsed intervertebral disc
  —Spinal osteochondritis
  —Juvenile chronic polyarthritis
  —Ankylosing spondylitis
  —Scoliosis
  —Reiter's disease
  —Nonspecific fatigue and depression

8
Backache in the middle-aged and elderly

Any cause of young backache may persist to cause trouble in middle or old age. Of the causes listed on page 62 much the most common are the traumatic, the mechanical and the degenerative. Osteoporosis is more common in the elderly. Psychogenic causes, including depression, may occur at any age.

Most older patients who complain of backache have few physical signs, no neurological signs and a poor localization of their discomfort. X-rays show no abnormality apart from degenerative changes which may or may not be relevant. This leaves the doctor to base his diagnosis on guesswork after taking account of the history, his assessment of the historian and a few physical signs, if any. The commoner causes of backache are those listed in group 1 of the Table overleaf. Most of the rest are rare, apart from those listed in group 5 – the psychogenic.

In a survey reported from the United States 50 per cent of sufferers from depression complained of pains in bones and joints and 80 per cent of this group had backache as their chief complaint. Depression alone can cause pain, or so it is said, but all of us have some spinal discomfort from time to time and depression, anxiety or other spiritual distress may fix on such an occasional disturbance, magnify it and perpetuate it.

EXAMINATION OF THE SPINE

There are some practical points in examination of the spine. Movements may be restricted in certain directions only and the pain may only be referred to certain segments. This suggests a local cause such as a disc protrusion, while the restriction of all movements in all directions suggests severe pain, great apprehension or a more diffuse involvement of the spine as in ankylosing spondylitis. Local tenderness on pressing firmly on the vertebral spines may help to localize a spinal disorder but it may be misleading in patients with a low pain threshold. This examination should be carried out with the patient lying on his abdomen, well relaxed and with his arms at his sides.

With the patient standing up, observe his stance and posture and ask him to demonstrate the movements of which he is capable. Touching the toes is an unreliable test of spinal flexion because ability to do this also depends on the mobility of the hips

Causes of chronic backache

1. Traumatic, structural, mechanical or degenerative
a) Low back strain: fatigue, obesity
b) Injuries of ligament, bone or joint
c) Osteoarthrosis
d) Intervertebral disc lesions
e) Instability syndromes (eg, spondylolisthesis)
f) Spinal stenosis
g) Congenital spinal abnormalities.

2. Metabolic
a) Osteomalacia
b) Osteoporosis
c) Ochronosis
d) Hyperparathyroidism
e) Fluorosis
f) Hypophosphataemia, rickets.

3. Unknown aetiology
a) Ankylosing spondylitis
b) The ankylosing spondylarthropathies
c) Osteochondritis
d) Paget's disease of bone.

4. Infective conditions affecting spine
a) Tuberculous disease
b) Undulant fever (abortus, melitensis)
c) Salmonella infections (eg, typhoid)
d) Syphilis
e) Yaws
f) Abscess (osteomyelitis).

5. Psychogenic
a) Anxiety
b) Depression
c) Compensation neurosis
d) Nondisease (malingering)
e) Hysteria.

6. Neoplastic, spinal and paraspinal
a) Malignant: Primary or secondary
carcinoma
Sarcoma
Multiple myeloma
Meningioma
Glioma
Reticuloses, eg, Hodgkin's disease
b) Benign: Neurofibroma.

7. Cardiac and vascular
a) Subarachnoid or spinal haemorrhage
b) Syphilitic or dissecting aneurysm
c) Grossly enlarged left atrium in mitral stenosis.

8. Gynaecological
a) Tuberculous disease
b) Chronic salpingitis
c) Chronic cervicitis
d) Tumours
e) Prolapsed or retroverted uterus (rarely)
f) Very large ovarian cyst (rarely).

9. Gastro-intestinal
a) Peptic ulcers
b) Cholelithiasis
c) Pancreatitis
d) Intra-abdominal new growth (colon, stomach, pancreas).

10. Renal
a) Carcinoma kidney
b) Calculus
c) Hydronephrosis
d) Polycystic kidney
e) Perinephric abscess
f) Prostatic neoplasm or abscess
g) Pyelonephritis, pyelitis
h) Renal medullary necrosis (necrotizing papillitis).

11. Blood disorders
a) Sickle cell crisis
b) Acute haemolytic crisis.

12. Drugs
a) Corticosteroids
b) Methysergide
c) Compound analgesic pills.

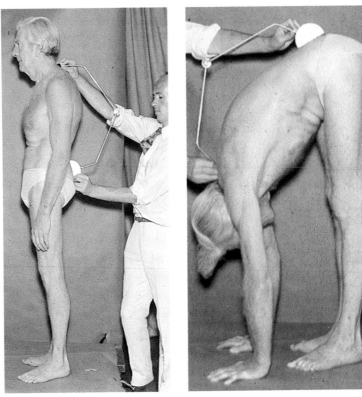

Figure 34 Measuring spinal flexion with Dunham's spondylometer.

and the length of the arms and legs. Spinal flexion can be measured with a spondylometer or an inclinometer. Loebl's inclinometer, which is a pendulum goniometer, can be obtained from the British Back Pain Association and has the advantage of being able to measure lateral movements of the spine as well as flexion and extension. In the absence of a special instrument, make two marks on the skin, one 10 cm above the lumbosacral junction and another 5 cm below this point in the erect posture. Then ask the patient to flex his spine as fully as possible and measure the distance between the two marks when he is in this position. The difference between the two measurements indicates the degree of flexion in this part of the spine.

A great deal can be learned by watching the patient move, undress, get on the couch, sit and stand, particularly if he does not know he is being observed. During further examination look for muscle wasting – which should be measured if possible – particularly in the calf and thigh, neurological signs as outlined in the Table on page 59, sensory changes, and alterations in tendon reflexes.

IMPORTANT CAUSES OF MIDDLE-AGED AND ELDERLY BACKACHE

Common spinal causes of backache

Back strain and postural fatigue are usually suggested by the history: certain activities or periods of prolonged immobility in unnatural postures lead to pain at the time or shortly afterwards.

Disc lesions   The history may be very suggestive, as when severe pain occurs with lightning rapidity on bending to lift a heavy weight. Such lesions are often accompanied by localizing neurological symptoms and signs.

Vertebral crush fractures occur more frequently in women than in men because osteoporosis is common in women after the menopause. The pain is severe and sudden in onset, localized to one area of the spine, often with tenderness on pressure over that area.

Multiple myeloma may present with severe bone pain in the back or elsewhere. A high ESR should lead one to order X-rays and blood examination for abnormal proteins. Bence-Jones proteinuria may be found.

Secondary malignant deposits   The most common primary sites are the breast in women and the bronchus in men.

Spinal stenosis

The spinal canal may be narrowed during development or by acquired disease. It may be narrowed centrally or laterally, damaging the nervous tissue directly or by leaving less space for it from protrusion of osteophytes or prolapsed discs – a combination of congenital (developmental) and acquired factors. The blood supply to the cauda equina may be affected, causing weakness, numbness or burning on exertion, that is eased by sitting and flexing the back but not by standing still. This condition resembles intermittent claudication (see Table opposite) but the abnormal sensations are felt in back, thigh and legs rather than in the calves only; calf cramps are absent; and peripheral pulses are present.

   Patients with spinal stenosis are usually over fifty years old and have a long history of backache, often with recent development of sciatica. The diagnosis is often made at operation although it may be revealed by special radiological techniques.

Reiter's disease

While Reiter's disease in childhood may be due to dysentery, in later life it is usually due to venereal infection. In either case it usually manifests itself after an interval of seven to ten days, sometimes with the classical triad of urethritis, conjunctivitis and arthritis. More often the conjunctivitis is absent, or so mild and transient that it is overlooked.

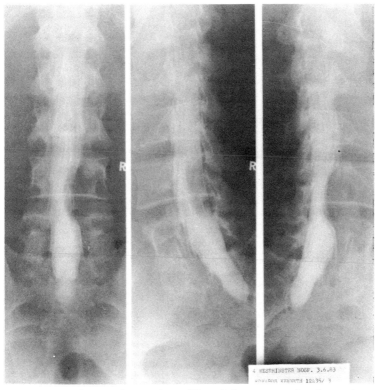

Figure 35 Myelogram showing large filling defect associated with spinal stenosis.

Whether Reiter's disease is due to dysentery or to venereal infection, the arthritis is usually peripheral and affects the lower more often than the upper limbs, but about 12 per cent of patients go on to develop ankylosing spondylitis with its typical sacro-iliac changes, after an interval of three to six years or even longer.

Intermittent claudication	Spinal stenosis
● Peripheral pulses absent in legs	● Peripheral pulses present in legs
● Cramps in calves in walking	● Weakness, numbness and burning in back and legs on walking
● Pains eased by standing still	● Pains eased by sitting or flexing spine
● Walking a set distance aggravates, worse uphill	● Walking uphill better than downhill
● Lumbar extension no effect	● Lumbar extension aggravates
● No bowel or bladder symptoms	● Bowel and bladder symptoms (pseudo-prostatism)

Mucocutaneous lesions may occur in the mouth in the early stages of either variety of Reiter's disease or on the penis in the venereal variety. The venereal variety may follow a gonococcal infection but there is usually a nonspecific urethritis from which none of the usual pathogens can be isolated, though 40 per cent are probably due to chlamydia trachomatis, 40 per cent to urea plasma urealyticum.

Inflammatory bowel disease

This may be followed by ankylosing spondylitis without the development of Reiter's disease. The victims are usually male. The ulcerative colitis or Crohn's disease which gave rise to the condition may be so mild that it is overlooked. The patients are usually $HLAB_{27}$ positive.

Psoriatic arthritis

This occurs in middle and old age but may also occur in adolescence or early adult life (see Chapter 20). It tends to occur around puberty as an asymmetrical peripheral arthritis in either sex, a minority progressing to ankylosing spondylitis. Ansell[1] noted that 42 per cent of her patients were $HLAB_{W17}$ and 25 per cent were $HLAB_{27}$ positive, correlating closely with the development of sacro-iliitis. There is often a family history of psoriasis. It is of interest that those patients who develop ankylosing spondylitis, either primarily or as part of psoriatic, colitic or Reiter's arthritis, tend to be $HLAB_{27}$ positive.

Spondylolysis and spondylolisthesis

A separation of the pars interarticularis (spondylolysis) may permit one vertebra to slip forward on another (spondylolisthesis). Backache may result but sometimes only on exertion or in full spinal flexion and in some cases the condition causes no symptoms.

A retired senior colleague, a famous athlete in his day, used to visit me at the Westminster Hospital when he had a complaint that interfered with his activities which included running in the park. On one occasion he complained of low backache that only afflicted him when he was doing a morning exercise that involved lying on his back and touching the wall behind his head with his feet, fully flexing his spine in the form of a letter C. The discomfort only occurred at this time, never when he ran. X-rays showed spondylolisthesis of L4 on L5 with about 1 cm displacement. When he omitted this particular exercise the symptoms ceased. Other patients are less fortunate and suffer severe and continuous pain for a time, but even though the deformity persists symptoms eventually abate, although they may recur with certain activities or exercises.

Spondylolysis and spondylolisthesis may be congenital, inborn anomalies of the upper sacrum or the arch of L5 allowing the displacement to occur, the lowest free lumbar vertebra slipping forward, usually during adolescence. The commonest predisposing lesion in the sacrum includes imperfect development of the inter-articular facets of L5 and S1. Spina bifida may be present in the same area. The developmental defect is said to be commoner in boys than in girls.

Bony lesions

A lytic lesion may occur in the pars articularis as a fatigue fracture. This may occur at any age but is rare under five. It is the commonest cause under the age of fifty and occurs more frequently in certain families. It is particularly common in female gymnasts. Over the age of fifty the commonest predisposing cause is degenerative change, more often at L4 than at L3 or L5, with a higher incidence in women. The discs and ligaments degenerate to allow overmobility in the area with facet degeneration and spondylolisthesis on the vertebra below.

Trauma may produce fractures in other areas such as facet or pedicle, leading to instability and local disease. Tuberculosis, Paget's disease or malignant growth may do the same. A lesion of the pars interarticularis is associated with backache in some but by no means in all cases. In one large study by MacNab[2] the lesion was found in 7.6 per cent of patients with backache and 7.6 per cent of people with no symptoms. When the patients were divided according to age it seemed that over forty years of age the incidence was the same as in the general population and that the lesion probably had little or nothing to do with the backache, while below the age of twenty-six the lesion was more likely to be the cause of the backache. Symptomatic treatment is adequate in most cases and surgery is very rarely needed.

Intra-abdominal causes of backache

Disease in the abdomen or pelvis may cause backache (see Table on page 62) and we must not forget our teachers' advice to make a pelvic examination in every case. The conditions listed in sections 7–10 of the Table are in fact rare as causes of backache and gynaecological disorders such as retroversion or prolapse of the uterus are very seldom the reason for severe or persistent backache.

Certain past cases of backache spring to mind: a tuberculous endometritis and salpingitis, a pelvic abscess, a carcinoma of the colon, a prostatic abscess, one syphilitic aneurysm of the aorta and two dissecting aneurysms that eroded spinal structures, both causing intolerable back pain which led one of the sufferers to suicide. In a satellite-mediated transatlantic quiz between Great Britain and the United States the British team won when they made the correct diagnosis that backache was being caused by a grossly enlarged left atrium in a patient with mitral disease.

WHAT TO DO

Avoiding aggravating factors

If there is no evidence of malignancy or any other cause outside the spine, the first recourse is to seek for causative or aggravating factors in the patient's life at work or at home. A badly designed chair at a table that is too high or too low may cause the spine to be held in a strained position all day long; car seats are often unsatisfactory; many people stand for work which could be done just as efficiently if they were sitting down; and sagging mattresses allow the spine to assume faulty positions during sleep. Gentle mobility is important, as in a rocking chair, and positions should be moved fairly frequently throughout the day so that unnatural positions are not held for long periods.

Employers should be encouraged to eliminate the need for work in bent or crouching positions, in confined spaces and on irregular surfaces. Many injuries and much chronic strain are caused by lifting heavy weights with the spine flexed: the spine and arms should be kept straight and leverage should take place at the knees and hips.

Home treatment, phase 1: Rest

A person with severe backache should rest, with analgesics and sedatives if necessary (see also Chapter 29 and 32). The beginning of rest should not be delayed until the condition has been aggravated by persistence in unsuitable activity. A few days of strict bed rest will often abort an attack of pain that would otherwise lead to weeks or months of painful incapacity. Rest often fails as a remedy because it is incomplete. If it is interrupted by getting out of bed to go to the lavatory, front door, telephone and kitchen it is not bed rest and will confer no benefit.

Most strains and soft tissue injuries will settle in a few days but more severe backache will probably need two to three weeks. There should be a commode in the bedroom and meals should be brought to the bedside. This is often difficult to arrange but other members of the family are more likely to try to make it possible if they can realize that bed rest is a form of treatment, not just an escape into idleness.

Home treatment, phase 2: Mobilization

Phase 2 includes gently increasing mobilization and exercise and home physiotherapy using hot showers, electric pads, heat in any convenient form and gentle exercises that increase as improvement proceeds.

Braces or belts may be used by patients who feel happier with a support. Some people like a woolly 'roll-on' for the lumbar spine. Others dislike any form of support and this attitude is usually to be encouraged because a belt or brace often becomes the symbol of an incapacity that no longer exists but is not easily forgotten.

Later treatment may include physiotherapy at a hospital or clinic with more exercises, possibly in a deep pool.

Treatment of minor backaches

These afflict every one of us at some time of our lives and they usually respond to modifications of behaviour, changes of furniture or car, simple analgesics or NSAIDs, physiotherapy, braces and belts or manipulation. It is only necessary to resort to bed rest (see Chapter 32) if the symptoms get worse or if there is no improvement in two or three weeks.

Treatment of resistant and persistent cases

Useful treatments are traction, manipulation or, in a few cases, extradural injection of large volumes of dilute local anaesthetic and a long-acting corticosteroid. Smaller amounts of anaesthetic and steroid may help when injected into painful or trigger spots.

Surgery

This is needed for relatively few backaches associated with disc protrusion and degenerative changes but it is indicated if severe pain persists in spite of full conservative treatment and particularly if there is persistence or advance of neurological signs. Lesions of the cauda equina with bowel or bladder involvement require urgent surgical decompression.

The best neurological and orthopaedic surgeons usually have the longest hospital waiting lists and this allows most severe backaches to recover while the patient is still waiting to be seen. Even when there is evidence of root pressure most cases settle with conservative treatment and if proper bed rest is not possible at home the patient should be admitted to hospital where even very severe backache will usually settle within three or four weeks.

Drugs

Drugs for severe backaches include analgesics and sedatives. Paracetamol 1 g tds or qds may be combined with diazepam 2–5 mg tds and nitrazepam 5–10 mg at night. Stronger analgesics (see Chapter 27) include dihydrocodeine (30–60 mg, 1–2 tablets, by mouth), buprenorphine 0.2–0.4 mg (1–2 tablets sublinqually), or if necessary Diconal (dipipanone 10 mg and cyclizine hydrochloride 30 mg, 1 tablet by mouth once or twice daily for 2–3 days only), or intramuscular (im) injections of pentazocine 30–60 mg, buprenorphine 0.3–0.6 mg or dihydrocodeine 50 mg.

In some countries dihydrocodeine injections and Diconal are subject to the misuse of drugs legislation and should be reserved for very painful episodes.

Drugs for severe backache
- **Mild oral**
  —paracetamol + diazepam (in the day)
  —paracetamol + nitrazepam (at night)
- **Strong oral**
  —dihydrocodeine
  —buprenorphine
  —Diconal (dipipanone + cyclizine hydrochloride)
- **Strong intramuscular**
  —pentazocine
  —buprenorphine
  —dihydrocodeine

PRACTICAL POINTS

- Much can be learned about the condition of the patient's spine by observing his movements during the consultation.
- Causes of backache in the middle-aged and elderly include:
  —Disc lesions
  —Vertebral crush fractures
  —Multiple myeloma
  —Spinal stenosis
  —Reiter's disease
  —Inflammatory bowel disease
  —Psoriatic arthritis
  —Spondylolysis and spondylolisthesthis
  —Bony lesions
  —Abdominal and pelvic disease
- Management of most cases of backache is based on:
  —Avoidance of aggravating factors
  —Rest followed by gentle mobilization, including physiotherapy
  —In some cases supports
  —Simple analgesics or NSAIDs

9

The changing face of rheumatology: differential diagnosis

HISTORICAL BACKGROUND

Rheumatic diseases have changed their shape and form over the centuries. There is no doubt that new diseases do appear and that some old ones disappear. The evidence of skeletal remains affirms that osteoarthrosis has been with man and beast for thousands of years but rheumatoid arthritis may not be nearly so ancient. Some writers believe it has only existed for a few hundred years or less.

The great modern change has been in titles and in the physician's list of diseases that his patients are allowed to have. Half way through the last century Archibald Garrod[1] suggested 'rheumatoid arthritis' as a name for the inflammatory variety of arthritis which he distinguished from osteoarthritis, but the term did not find general use until many years later. Gout, rheumatism and arthritis made up the diagnostic ration of a hundred years ago and all the many other forms of arthropathy had to be compressed into one of these categories.

Gout

Gout was a popular favourite with physicians over the ages and took much more than its diagnostic fair share. There were gouty eczema, gouty iritis and every other sort of gouty arthritis, while in 1888 Bruce gave the name of 'senile rheumatic gout' to what we now call polymyalgia rheumatica (see Chapter 13).

In 1884 Arthur Conan Doyle, no less, wrote to tell the *Lancet* about a gentleman he had seen, a Mr H, who had what appeared to be eczema and psoriasis. Doyle gave him arsenic and potassium iodide without much benefit but remained content with his diagnosis until he saw Mr H's daughter, Mrs B, who came to him with pain in the eyes and indigestion. He then found that her grandfather, Mr H's father, had suffered from gout and the scales fell from his eyes. 'Recognizing this to be a gouty symptom and bethinking me of the obscure skin disease which affected the father . . .' he diagnosed nonarthritic gout and prescribed alkalies and colchicum. Father and daughter then rapidly improved. Sherlock Holmes might perhaps have done better but psoriatic arthropathy had not been described at this time so that even he would have had difficulties – and Dr Watson would have got nowhere.

Only a week earlier the famous Dr Jonathan Hutchinson FRS[2] had published his

Bowman Lecture in the same journal. He wrote of 'hot eyes, irritable eyes and quiet gout', and noted that 'arthritic iritis' might occur in gonorrhoeal rheumatism. He also described a lady who had crippling involvement of the terminal phalanges in association with 'destructive iritis'. Quite sure that this was gout, he opened one joint, expecting to find uratic material, but only obtained a soft, jelly-like substance. Even the best people could not diagnose conditions that had not been described or identified; and those three terms – rheumatism, arthritis and gout (or a gouty syndrome) – had to cover what are now known to be around 180 different conditions.

PROGRESS IN DIAGNOSTIC LABELLING

The physicians who tidied up the diagnostic field made most of their progress by clinical observation with careful follow up. Anklyosing spondylitis, psoriatic arthropathy, Reiter's (Brodie's) disease, polymyalgia rheumatica, giant cell arteritis, enteropathic arthritis and the several subdivisions of what used to be called Still's disease – now called juvenile chronic polyarthritis (JCP) – have all been identified within the last hundred years and most of them within the last three or four decades. Laboratory, X-ray and other ancillary techniques have been of immense help during the last forty years but the major reclassifications of disease have been based on clinical evidence, usually involving long follow up.

Ankylosing spondylitis

During the last forty years of the previous century French and English clinicians had noted that this disease occurred predominantly in young males and progressed as spinal stiffening, with peripheral joints affected infrequently and usually transiently. American physicians called this disease 'rheumatoid spondylitis' on the strength of nonspecific inflammatory histological changes in peripheral joints, but later work has shown the Europeans to have been right. The patients knew the difference all along and neither liked nor benefited from the rheumatoid therapy of rest and splintage: in fact very much the opposite. (See Chapter 32.)

Psoriatic arthropathy

It was noted that the arthropathy associated with psoriasis was more patchy than rheumatoid arthritis, and that it involved the terminal interphalangeal joints of the fingers and sometimes the spine where it resembled ankylosing spondylitis. Psoriasis can coexist with rheumatoid arthritis because they are both common, but psoriatic arthropathy differs in those clinical respects and rheumatoid factor remains absent from the serum. (See Chapter 20.)

Reiter's (Brodie's) disease

In 1818 Benjamin Brodie described four male patients who had developed polyarthritis, mostly of the lower extremities, with urethritis and conjunctivitis, all following venereal infection. It was not until ninety-eight years later, in 1916, that Hans Reiter described the same triad in a German cavalry officer. He thought this was a manifestation of spirochaetal infection. The same syndrome was soon reported from behind the French lines.

In 1940 an epidemic of Flexner dysentery among the Finns who were holding back the Russians was followed two weeks later by an outbreak of Reiter's disease. This postinfective condition recalled rheumatic fever in that the disease followed an acute infection after a latent period.

Polymyalgia rheumatica

Horton[3] described giant cell arteritis in the United States in the 1930s. Stewart Barber in Buxton (1957)[4] described a number of elderly patients who had morning stiffness and pain in the shoulder and hip girdle areas with a high erythrocyte sedimentation rate (ESR). This syndrome had already been noted but was considered to be a form of rheumatoid arthritis in the elderly. Barber followed up his patients for two to three years and found that they did not develop rheumatoid arthritis. He suggested that this should be regarded as a disease in its own right and proposed the name 'polymyalgia rheumatica'.

Once the idea had been scotched that these people were merely elderly rheumatoids and physicians looked at them in a fresh light as victims of a separate disorder, they began to get the attention and treatment they deserved. It later came to be appreciated that giant cell arteritis and polymyalgia rheumatica are probably two phases of the same disease and most rheumatologists hold this opinion today. (See Chapter 13.)

Other arthropathies

We learned that the association between arthritis and Crohn's disease and ulcerative colitis is more than a coincidence.

Barbara Ansell and Eric Bywaters[5] then showed, again as a result of careful clinical study and long follow up, that Still's disease (JCP) is usually something different from rheumatoid arthritis in a child and is, in fact, a separate seronegative arthritis with clinical features unlike those of adult rheumatoid disease. Only some 8 per cent of the children they studied eventually turned out to have rheumatoid arthritis. About 10 per cent, usually boys, went on to develop ankylosing spondylitis and a few showed some other disorder of connective tissue, but most remained as seronegative arthropathies. Still had originally held that the condition which he described at the Great Ormond Street Hospital in London was not rheumatoid arthritis and he seems to have been 92 per cent right. The careful clinical studies of Ansell and Bywaters proved the point.

Identification of systemic lupus erythematosus (SLE), mixed connective tissue disease and many other disorders has largely depended on laboratory criteria but most of the major diseases have crystallized out, as it were, on essentially clinical grounds. The Wassermann reaction distinguished syphilitic disorders and discovery of the tubercle bacillus accounted for tuberculous disease of bones and joints, but for many of the rest the patients themselves have often noted the essential differences between their conditions, even if these were not at the time so clear to their doctors.

Major characteristics of the more common arthropathies

Diagnosis	Characteristic features	Coexistent disorders	Investigation
Giant cell arteritis	Temporal headaches, tender inflamed arteries – typically temporal. Absent pulses, haemic murmurs. Patient usually over 60 years of age.		● SR 60+ in 1 hour. ● RF −ve.
Polymyalgia rheumatica	Pains and morning stiffness in shoulders and hips. Patient usually over 60 years of age.		● SR 60+ in 1 hour. ● RF −ve.
Psoriatic arthropathy	Patchy polyarthritis with terminal interphalangeal finger joints often involved. Sometimes spondylitis.	Psoriasis, sometimes slight. Nail beds often pitted, ridged or yellow (psoriasis).	● RF −ve.
Enteropathic arthropathy	Asymmetrical polyarthritis often associated with relapse of colitis. Knees affected 30%, ankles 50%, ankylosing spondylitis 5%.	Ulcerative colitis or Crohn's disease.	● RF −ve. ● biopsy +ve. ● Ba studies +ve.
Ankylosing spondylitis	Mostly young males. Stiffness and pain in spine and girdle joints (hips and shoulders). Iritis in 30%.		● RF −ve. ● HLA_{B27}+ in over 90% of cases. ● Sacro-iliac X rays +ve.
Systemic lupus erythematosus (SLE)	90% females. Very varied symptomatology – referred to any system. Patients often more ill than arthritic and often febrile.		● ANF +ve. ● SR raised. ● Anti-DNA +. ● Often anaemic. ● LE cells present.
Hydralazine syndrome	Drug-induced SLE caused by many other agents as well as hydralazine. Recovers on stopping drugs.		● LE tests revert to normal on stopping therapy.
Gout	Acute pain and swelling and redness in big toe/foot/ankle/knee. 90% males. Onset often at night.	Possibly polycythaemia or renal disease.	● Serum uric acid raised. ● Urate crystals in joint fluid.
Pyrophosphate arthropathy	Males = females. Knee commonest site. Acute pain and swelling.	Rarely hyperparathyroidism, haemochromatosis and hypophosphatasia.	● Pyrophosphate crystals in joint fluid. ● X rays often +ve.

Diagnosis	Characteristic features	Coexistent disorders	Investigation
Polymyositis	Muscle pains, weakness and tenderness. May be pains in joints with morning stiffness.		● Muscle biopsy +ve. ● EMG abnormal. ● Serum aldolase and other enzymes raised.
Dermatomyositis	Lilac hue features and fingers. Muscle weakness and tenderness.	Malignant disease often present in middle aged and elderly.	● Biopsy. ● Muscle enzymes. ● EMG.
Progressive systemic sclerosis (scleroderma)	Tight fingers, blanched fingers and face. Raynaud's syndrome, often dysphagia. More common in females.		● Biopsy.
Mixed connective tissue disease (MCTD)	Like scleroderma with features SLE and polymyostosis.		● ANF +ve. ● Ribonuclear protein antibodies +ve.
Polyarteritis nodosa	More common in males. Generalized muscle and joint aches. Fever, variable polyarthritis. Symptoms referred to any system – particularly musculo-skeletal, renal, pulmonary ('asthma') and neuropathy.		● Biopsy. ● Australia antigen may be present.
Rheumatoid arthritis	3:1 female to male ratio. Polyarthritis often starting metatarsal heads, fingers, wrists. Joints swollen, painful, stiff and tender, but fingertip joints usually spared.		● X rays +ve. ● RF +ve in 80% cases: early mild cases often−ve.
Osteoarthritis	One or several joints, hard and knobbly terminal finger joints, thumb bases, knees, big toes and hips commonest. Patients usually middle aged or elderly.	Old injury to joints may have been present (fracture or dislocation).	● ESR not raised above 30. ● RF −ve. ● X rays +ve.

THE FUTURE

It is likely that osteoarthrosis and rheumatoid arthritis will both fragment further in the future and throw off new clinical entities which will demand new therapeutic approaches. When some of the patients who are thought to be suffering from a particular disease have a different clinical form of disorder, with a different progression, a different age-sex incidence, a different prognosis and a different response to various basic forms of therapy we must ask ourselves whether we have a separate clinical entity that ought to be studied separately in its own right. The history of ankylosing spondylitis provides an outstanding example.

In the interest of further advance we must refrain from trying to force any 'anomalous' patient into a category which does not truly fit him and the follow up of these anomalies must be as long and meticulous as possible.

The Table on pages 74–5 lists the more important characteristics of the commoner arthropathies.

All the above, with the exception of osteoarthrosis, may have raised ESR and anaemia. Rheumatoid factor is diagnostic of rheumatoid arthritis if the clinical features of the disease are present, but it may also be present, though rarely, in normal people, in chronic hepatitis, in tropical illnesses such as malaria and kala-azar, in bacterial endocarditis, SLE, scleroderma, polymyositis, dermatomyositis and some other conditions. In Europeans with arthritic symptoms and signs a titre of 1/64 or higher is usually diagnostic of rheumatoid arthritis.

10
Arthritis in the elderly

BACKGROUND

Rheumatic disorders are common in old age: much of rheumatology is geriatric and much of geriatrics is rheumatological. Osteoarthrosis, for instance, is common in old age but because degenerative changes are present in all elderly subjects care is needed in differential diagnosis. The symptoms complained of may have nothing to do with those degenerative changes but may be due to another, coexisting disorder.

It has been said that perhaps 12 per cent of the population between the ages of sixty-five and sixty-nine have a significant disability and that the incidence of such disability increases to reach 80 per cent at the age of eighty, a significant disability being defined as a state in which it is impossible to exist at home without help. One quarter of these disabled people have severe joint disease.[1]

Of the four great afflictions of old age – immobility, falls, mental confusion and incontinence – the first two are often directly due to locomotor disease.

Rheumatoid arthritis, ankylosing spondylitis and the other various seronegative arthropathies become less common although their effects persist in those who have survived.

Osteoporosis, osteoarthrosis and polymyalgia rheumatica become more common as the years go by.

The older patient is less inclined to complain and may consult his doctor less frequently, partly because he has learned to live with his disability which he accepts as inevitable, and partly because he may regard the possible therapeutic reward as unlikely to repay the effort required to obtain it. Treatment is made more difficult by the fact that an older body's ability to handle drugs is often impaired and tolerance may be lower than in the younger age groups.

OSTEOARTHROSIS IN THE ELDERLY

Osteoarthrosis takes many different forms. It is usual to divide it into primary and secondary types but so-called primary osteoarthrosis probably includes several different entities.

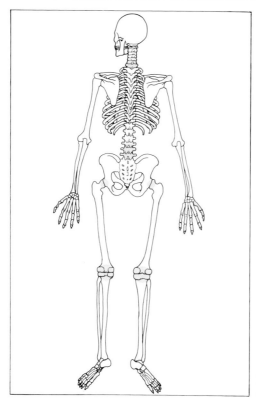

Figure 36 Sites most commonly affected by osteoarthrosis.

Secondary osteoarthrosis

This occurs in areas previously damaged by injury, disease or congenital abnormality as:

1. **A local monarthrosis** affecting only one joint, as after a fracture, dislocation, haemarthrosis, pyarthrosis, avascular necrosis, acetabular dysplasia of the hip or inversion of the acetabular labrum. The cause of a monarthrosis may also affect another neighbouring joint but this is essentially a local lesion.
2. **A general, polyarticular condition** following inflammatory polyarthritis, infective arthritis or a haemorrhagic state.

Apparently primary osteoarthrosis

This usually takes a polyarticular form as in the common generalized postmenopausal osteoarthrosis described by Kellgren and Moore in Manchester in 1952.[2] There are other varieties of primary polyarticular osteoarthrosis and I have seen several severely affected patients with normal peripheral and intermediate joints and no Heberden's nodes but with extensive osteoarthrotic changes throughout the cervical and lumbar spines and in both hips.

Diagnostic difficulties

Osteoarthrosis is frequently misdiagnosed because most elderly people have some degenerative changes in the joints and it is easy to ascribe the symptoms of another organic disease to those degenerative changes. Coexisting conditions that are liable to be overlooked include:

- Polymyalgia rheumatica
- Paget's disease of bone
- Hyperparathyroidism
- Myxoedema
- Myeloma
- Primary or secondary malignant disease of bone
- Pseudohypertrophic pulmonary osteoarthropathy
- Avascular necrosis
- Chondrocalcinosis
- Osteomalacia
- Osteoporosis with crush fractures

Psychiatric conditions are common in the elderly and the symptoms of depression or anxiety state may wrongly be attributed to joint changes which have been revealed by X-rays. Sometimes there is no organic or classifiable psychiatric disorder but the patient is unhappy and discontented and wishes for more sympathy and attention. Symptoms that are truly an emotional appeal for greater kindness are liable, in such cases, to be attributed to any degenerative changes that happen to have been discovered.

Differential diagnosis

While there is no disorder of adults that cannot coexist with osteoarthrosis, those which are most likely to cause diagnostic confusion are:

Paget's disease of bone   X-ray findings are typical and the serum alkaline phosphatase is raised. Paget's disease is usually symptomless but there may be acute painful episodes, sometimes due to tiny fractures in the areas of condensed bone. It is possible that there are vascular causes for some acutely painful incidents.

Polymyalgia rheumatica, with or without localizing signs of giant cell arteritis, usually occurs in people over sixty, all of whom have degenerative changes in bones and joints, but the onset of new and quite different symptoms should warn the physician that something new and quite different has started to happen. The patient is quite accustomed to his osteoarthrotic symptoms but now has pains in the neck, shoulder and hip which are worse in the early morning and often fail to ease until midday

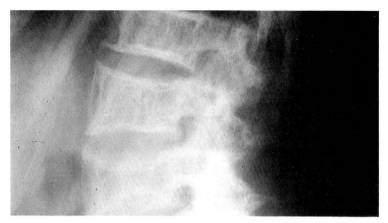

Figure 37   Typical Paget's disease in lumbar vertebrae of an elderly lady.

(polymyalgia rheumatica) or local tenderness over certain arteries such as the temporals (giant cell arteritis). The patient now starts to use such adjectives as 'excruciating' or 'agonizing', and it should soon become clear that these pains are something new and different from the milder symptoms of his long-established osteoarthrosis.

Endocrine disorders   There are three endocrine disorders that may be confused with osteoarthrosis.

1. **Diabetic amyotrophy** is more common in men. A reversible muscle weakness of the thighs may masquerade as osteoarthrosis of the hips or knees.
2. **Myxoedema** is usually obvious. Early or doubtful cases can be verified by serological estimation of thyroid hormones.
3. **Hyperparathyroidism** may cause osteitis fibrosa cystica. The serum alkaline phosphatase is raised and X-rays may suggest the diagnosis by showing cystic or other bone changes.

Spinal conditions   Spondylolisthesis, osteoporosis and osteomalacia are often found in elderly arthritic subjects but are commoner in women. There is gradual bone loss after the age of forty-five in women and fifty-five in men but it is unusual for symptoms to occur before the age of sixty to seventy in either sex. Sudden severe pain in an osteoporotic spine suggests a crush fracture of a vertebral body.

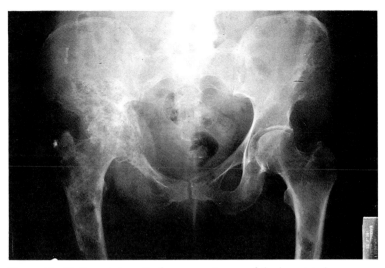

Figure 38 Malignant deposits from a carcinoma of the breast in bones around the right hip, presenting like a case of osteoarthrosis, with pain and stiffness localized to this joint and no loss of weight or systemic upset.

Malignant deposits in bone may cause no symptoms or may manifest themselves with pains or fractures in spine, pelvis or elsewhere. In pseudohypertrophic pulmonary osteoarthropathy, usually but by no means always due to a carcinoma of the bronchus, the patient's condition may resemble an inflammatory arthritis rather than osteoarthrosis, with effusions in ankles and/or knees, but clubbing of fingers and radiological evidence of new bone formation under the periosteum in forearms and lower legs are usually present as pointers to the true diagnosis. The most common primary sites for bone secondaries are bronchus and prostate in men and breast in women, but other primary growths, including those of thyroid, may also metastasize to bone. Sarcoma sometimes appears years after radiotherapy for some other condition or in Paget's disease but primary sarcoma of bone is rare in old age. Myeloma is easily overlooked but may appear in many forms in people over forty, ranging from diffuse aches and local pains in the spine, thorax or pelvis to a sudden agonizing backache. Dermatomyositis is rare in old age and its occurrence suggests an underlying malignant condition.

The ageing process

As people grow older they suffer a diminution of energy and vigour with a lessening of libido and sexual potency and of appetites of all types except, in many cases, for alcohol and tobacco. There is a decline and slowing of many bodily functions including those of the liver and kidneys. Older people are inclined to do less and rest more so that they become stiffer and less mobile, and their muscles grow weaker. They may suffer pain, loss of consciousness, and drop attacks in which they fall to the ground without warning (see Chapter 22). Memory for recent events becomes poorer and the lack of anything to look forward to increases their tendency to be apathetic and self-centred. Spinal osteoporosis increases but there is thickening and remoulding of bone around osteoarthrotic joints where the bones become denser rather than more rarified. Arterial sclerosis in myocardium, brain and legs may combine to reduce the capacity for exertion.

So it is that many osteoarthrotic patients who do not complain directly of joint symptoms tend to do less, go out less often and adopt a diminished lifestyle that is dictated by the gradual failure of all their physiological systems. Improvement of the condition may be brought about by a carefully monitored programme of rest and exercise (see Chapter 32).

RHEUMATOID ARTHRITIS

Rheumatoid arthritis which started in early or middle age may cease to be active during the later years although the structural damage it has caused remains, on which is superimposed the degenerative changes of old age. Rheumatoid arthritis may, however, begin after the age of sixty-five and may present in one of three ways:

1. Insidiously and gradually in a few or several joints.
2. As an acute polyarthritis in several joints.
3. In girdles (shoulders and hips), masquerading as polymyalgia rheumatica (see Chapter 13).

In a recent survey of the literature Fox[3] notes that when rheumatoid arthritis begins in old age it tends to be milder and less deforming, although there are exceptions to this rule.[4] Extra-articular manifestations, apart from anaemia, are less common, and the female preponderance is less marked than in the younger age groups. Fox states that in Great Britain levels of rheumatoid factor in the blood of 1 in 128 can be taken as diagnostic of rheumatoid arthritis in the elderly but that lower levels are questionable.

Once the diagnosis has been made treatment (see also Chapter 28) is on the same lines as for younger people with three important differences:

1. Multiple diagnoses are common.
2. Rehabilitation, both physical and psychological, may be more difficult and have to be applied more gently.
3. Drug treatment is more hazardous.

SERONEGATIVE ARTHROPATHIES

These conditions rarely start in old age and are likely to have persisted from an earlier time of life. The older patient with ankylosing spondylitis, psoriatic arthritis or colitic arthropathy, for example, has probably had his or her disorder for many years. Treatment, apart from the difficulties just mentioned, is on the same lines as for younger patients. Reiter's disease occasionally if rarely persists into old age as a mon- or pauciarticular arthritis.

PRESCRIBING FOR THE ELDERLY ARTHRITIS SUFFERER

Much has been written about prescribing for children but little, until recently, about prescribing for the aged. The current British National Formulary,[5] however, does point out that many older people exhibit deterioration of body systems, metabolic deficiencies and multiple pathological processes, and that the number of adverse effects is therefore comparatively high in this age group. Special care is needed when several physicians are prescribing for several different maladies.

Compliance is often poor and self-medication is common. Overmedication is a frequent reason for the admission of older people to hospital but many others have to be admitted for undermedication, a common example being the aged sufferer from heart disease who has failed to take his diuretic.

Because a broken neck of femur is often a death sentence for an old and osteoporotic subject it is necessary to take great care when giving any drug which may befuddle or oversedate, particularly at night. The fewer and simpler the medicines and the less often they have to be taken, the more likely it is that an old person will use them as the doctor intends.

Liver function

This may be impaired in old age but the hepatic reserve is usually large enough to metabolize most drugs efficiently, even if the patient is taking too much alcohol. Hypoproteinaemia, however, is common in the inflammatory arthropathies as well as being a feature of the ageing process. It is therefore important to be cautious in the use of drugs which may compete with one another for protein-binding sites and such drugs include all the NSAIDs, warfarin, prednisone and other corticosteroids and phenytoin. Existing routine liver function tests are a poor guide to the ability of a liver to deal with most drugs.

Renal function

This declines with age and since many drugs and their metabolites are excreted in the urine the efficiency of the kidneys should be checked before administration of a drug whose elimination depends on them. A glomerular filtration rate of less than 10 ml/min with a serum creatinine over 700 mmol per litre indicates severely diminished renal function.

Certain of the long-term anti-inflammatory drugs, including gold salts and penicil- lamine, are potentially nephrotoxic while the NSAIDs inhibit prostaglandin synthetase and may so produce oedema or lessen the action of diuretics, phenylbutazone being an example.

According to Braverman[6] elderly people are exceptionally liable to unwanted gastrointestinal and dermatological effects of drugs while Inman[7] noted that aplastic anaemia as a complication of treatment with phenylbutazone or oxyphenbutazone was six times as common in women aged over sixty-five as in any other age-sex group. Cooke and Thomson[8] and Gleeson[9] found older women particularly prone to peptic-ulcer provocation by NSAIDs.

PRACTICAL POINTS

● Maintain greatest possible mobility, morale and interest in the world in general.
● Whenever possible treat the patient at home: old people generally react badly to a change of environment.
● Keep physical and occupational therapy within realistic bounds that the patient can easily tolerate.
● Give positive rather than negative advice: do's rather than don'ts.
● Give as few drugs as seldom as possible and select them with regard to individual renal, gastrointestinal, haemopoietic and CNS capacity as well as to any other drugs the patient may be taking.
● Be sure that the patient understands what he is supposed to be doing and taking, and when, recheck this frequently and do everything possible to ensure compliance.

11
Juvenile chronic polyarthritis

Juvenile chronic polyarthritis (JCP), also called Still's disease, is not a common condition – a general practitioner may expect a new case every fifteen years. But once it has appeared JCP is a persistently chronic disorder requiring many years of care, with closest collaboration between general practice, community services and the hospital. It does, however, have a surprisingly good prognosis.

Although there had been isolated reports of polyarthritis in children before 1897 it was the masterly description by George Frederick Still, when a medical registrar at the Hospital for Sick Children, Great Ormond Street, London, that put JCP on the medical map. He gave an excellent account of the disease in its acute and chronic forms and noted that it was different from adult polyarthritis. To this day, however, in many parts of the world, the disease described by Still is misnamed as 'juvenile rheumatoid arthritis'.

Still described twenty-two cases in all, twelve of whom had splenomegaly, lymphadenopathy and fever. He noted involvement of pleura and pericardium but did not mention the characteristic rash.

CLINICAL FEATURES

My own interest in the condition started in 1935 when I was working as house physician and then registrar at the Royal Northern Hospital, London, under Dr Bernard Schlesinger of Great Ormond Street. He was particularly interested in polyarthritis and rheumatic fever in children. It was then that I came to recognize that the essential features of JCP are:

1. **Inflammatory arthritis** affecting a few or many joints, including the interphalangeal joints of the fingers. Five or more joints are affected in about half of the cases, four or fewer in the rest.
2. **Lymph-node enlargement** in about 50 per cent.
3. **Splenomegaly** in about 25 per cent.
4. **Fever**, often high and intermittent at first. There is a febrile onset in about 33 per cent. It responds to salicylates but not to antibacterials.

5. **Subcutaneous nodules** in only about 10 per cent. They usually have the acute, soft appearance and feel of the nodules that are found in rheumatic fever.
6. **A maculopapular rash**, often transient, in about a third.
7. **Transient pericarditis or pleurisy** in 10 per cent or more.
8. **Iritis** in about 11 per cent. This sometimes leads to band opacities of the cornea and occasionally to cataracts.
9. **The cervical spine** is often involved and may become fixed and rigid.
10. **Growth** is affected. The child is smaller than usual, with the 'sparrow jaw' or underdeveloped mandible that causes a receding chin and a bird-like appearance.
11. **Amyloidosis** in 2–8 per cent.
12. **Rheumatoid factor** is only found in around 10 per cent.

Who gets it?

Juvenile chronic polyarthritis occurs slightly more often in girls. It usually starts between two and four, and eleven and thirteen years of age.

CLASSIFICATION AND DIAGNOSIS

At a 1977 meeting under the auspices of the European League against Rheumatism (EULAR) and the World Health Organisation (WHO) it was agreed that a diagnosis of JCP ought only to be made if the disease began before the age of sixteen and lasted at least three months.

Cases were to be classified by mode of onset as:

1. Systemic illness.
2. Polyarthritis.
3. Pauciarticular (four or fewer joints).

Dr Barbara Ansell, who reports the EULAR-WHO criteria, followed 161 cases for over 15 years and reported (1971) that in JCP:

● 106 remained seronegative
● 27 had developed ankylosing spondylitis
● 23 had juvenile rheumatoid arthritis
● 4 had psoriatic arthritis
● 1 remained uncertain.[1]

Other arthritides

There is a present tendency for every arthritic child to be diagnosed as suffering from JCP but it must be remembered that there are other, if rarer, causes of arthritis in children, including the arthritis associated with ulcerative colitis and Crohn's disease (regional enteritis), systemic lupus erythematosus, polyarteritis nodosa, scleroderma, rheumatic fever, post-dysenteric arthritis and postdysenteric Reiter's disease, poly-myositis and dermatomyositis.

Mimics

It is also necessary to exclude conditions which may mimic JCP: haemophilia, leukaemia, pyarthrosis, vasculitis in Henoch-Schönlein purpura, Behçet's disease, sickle cell disease, thalassaemia, tropical disorders such as kala-azar and plant-thorn arthritis (a granulomatous inflammation, usually found in the knee, caused by penetration of a joint by a thorn, a sharp grass-blade or other vegetable matter).

Many children who are growing fast in early adolescence experience 'growing pains' for which there is no ready explanation.

A malignant growth may be found: for instance neuroblastoma involving and penetrating the bone.

Trauma and congenital abnormalities, such as hypermobility syndrome in 'double-jointed' children, and dietetic deficiencies such as scurvy and rickets all have to be considered.

Quite apart from organic disease a large number of 'functional' conditions may be associated with arthralgia: they have many causes, from hard, uncomfortable boots to a desire to avoid school.

The Table overleaf outlines the larger diagnostic field. While most of the conditions listed are very rare they must be kept in mind when the diagnosis is uncertain. In many cases the correct diagnosis will only be revealed by follow up for several weeks, months or even years.

Likely types

In developed countries today the more common chronic polyarthropathies found in children under the age of sixteen are probably JCP, juvenile ankylosing spondylitis, juvenile rheumatoid arthritis and leukaemia. Many of the conditions listed in the Table cause joint pain (polyarthralgia) rather than true polyarthritis with physical signs in the joints, but they may, nevertheless, cause diagnostic confusion.

CLINICAL GROUPS

JCP falls roughly into three groups, systemic, polyarticular and pauciarticular.

1. Systemic

This variety affects about one-third of the patients. The onset of the disease is with remittent fever, high in the evening, slightly raised or normal in the morning. A transient erythematous rash accompanies the fever in about 40 per cent of cases. It is best seen on the trunk or limbs and is often precipitated by a hot bath. Generalized lymphadenopathy occurs in about 25 per cent and splenomegaly, hepatomegaly, pericarditis and pleurisy in 25 per cent or fewer. Abdominal pain, anaemia and weight loss are common but joint symptoms may be minimal at this stage, often taking several months to appear.

Polyarthritis and polyarthralgia in childhood

1. Primary connective tissue disorders
—Juvenile chronic arthritis (seronegative)
—Juvenile ankylosing spondylitis
—Juvenile rheumatoid arthritis (seropositive)
—Psoriatic arthritis
—Enteropathic arthritis (with Crohn's disease or ulcerative colitis)
—Systemic lupus erythematosus
— Progressive systemic sclerosis (scleroderma)
—Polymyositis and dermatomyositis
—Mixed connective tissue disease

2. Infective conditions
—Pyogenic (septic) arthritis
—Tuberculosis of bone and joint
—Viral arthropathies (as in rubella, mumps, chicken-pox, infective mononucleosis and infective hepatitis)
—Subacute bacterial endocarditis
—Brucellosis
—Meningococcal arthritis
—Syphilis (Clutton's joints)
—Plant-thorn arthritis
—Epidemic arthritis (eg, Lyme arthritis, Ross River fever)

3. Postinfective
—Rheumatic fever
—Reiter's syndrome
—Postdysenteric synovitis
—Jaccouds arthritis (postrheumatic fever)

4. Allergic conditions
—Serum sickness
—Henoch-Schönlein purpura

5. Haematological disorders
—Leukaemia
—Haemophilia
—Christmas disease
—Sickle cell disease
—Thalassaemia

6. Nutritional
—Scurvey
—Rickets

7. Neoplastic
—Lymphoma
—Neuroblastoma
—Histiocytoma

8. Immunodeficiency states
—Hypogammaglobulinaemia (Agammaglobulinaemia)
—Complement component deficiencies
—Selective IgA deficiency

9. Metabolic and congenital
—Mediterranean fever
—Lesch-Nyhan syndrome
—Familial hypercholesterolaemia
—Lipogranulomatosis (Farber's disease)
—Mucopolysaccharoidosis
—Gaucher's disease
—Hypermobility syndromes (eg, Ehlers-Danlos)

10. Trauma
—Bad footwear
—Injury
—Osteogenesis imperfecta

11. Tropical diseases
—Kala-azar
—Yaws
—Malaria

12. Psychogenic and nondisease
—Hysteria
—Behaviour disorders
—Functional and emotional upsets
—Malingering

13. Miscellaneous
—Sarcoidosis
—Osteochondritis
—Amyloidosis
—Chondromalacia patellae
—Growing pains

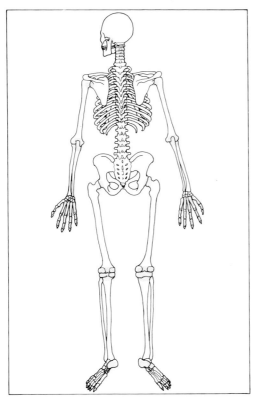

Figure 39 Sites more commonly affected in juvenile chronic polyarthritis.

2. Polyarticular

Joint symptoms of pain, swelling and stiffness may come on rapidly or gradually and either progress relentlessly or remit and relapse. Joint involvement is usually bilateral and symmetrical, affecting knees, small joints of hands and feet, wrists, ankles, elbows and jaws. Involvement of the neck is common. Hips are affected in about 40 per cent and this may be a major cause of crippling.

3. Pauciarticular

In this form from one to four joints are affected, usually the larger ones. Joint symptoms are rare but iridocyclitis is common and may cause band keratopathy, secondary glaucoma and cataracts at a later stage. This iridocyclitis is found in about 11 per cent of all cases, its first signs being a punctate precipitate on the posterior surface of the cornea (keratitis punctata or KP). This unpleasant feature of the disease often occurs with no symptoms at first and no outward sign of inflammation. It must therefore be sought for early and repeatedly. Slit lamp examination is necessary for this purpose. Patients in this group have a higher incidence of both iridocyclitis and antinuclear factor than those in other groups.

OTHER FORMS OF JUVENILE POLYARTHRITIS

Juvenile ankylosing spondylitis

This condition has been discussed in Chapter 7. It occurs six times more frequently in boys than in girls and is the only form of juvenile chronic arthritis to show a male predominance. In Ansell's series the mean age of onset was twelve years, the most common early symptoms arising from hips, knees and ankles. In only a minority was the onset polyarticular while only one patient had back pain as an early symptom. Ninety per cent were $HLAB_{27}$ positive. The average time taken to develop the typical sacro-iliac X-ray changes was five and a half years from onset of symptoms. The mean age at which limitation of back movement occurred was 19.8 years. Iridocyclitis did not occur initially but was found in nearly 25 per cent of cases at some time in the follow-up period.

Juvenile seropositive rheumatoid arthritis

This represents 8–10 per cent of cases of chronic polyarthritis in childhood and must be distinguished from seronegative Still's disease. It follows the adult pattern of rheumatoid arthritis quite closely with involvement of small joints of hands and feet, rheumatoid nodules being present in some 25 per cent. The course is longer and more severe than in seronegative disease and erosions are seen in X-rays at an earlier stage. IgM rheumatoid factor is positive within a few months of onset which occurs at the age of ten or later in 70 per cent of cases.

INVESTIGATIONS OF JCP

- **Normochromic and normocytic anaemia** with marked polymorphonuclear leucocytosis is common.
- **The ESR** is usually raised unless only one joint is involved.
- **The immunoglobulins** may be diffusely raised but a more common finding is a moderate increase of IgG only.
- **Antinuclear factor** is present in 30 per cent of cases and is associated with iridocyclitis in 85 per cent of these.
- **Anti-DNA antibodies and rheumatoid factor** are both absent.
- **Radiological changes** may develop later: periarticular osteoporosis around affected joints and of phalanges adjacent to flexor tendon involvement are the earliest. There may be premature appearance of epiphyses in young children and premature fusion in older ones. Erosions are late or absent in JCP, in contrast to juvenile rheumatoid arthritis where they occur earlier and more commonly.

COMPLICATIONS

Growth defects

These may be general or local, affecting jaw, neck or leg. Severe disease with considerable metabolic upset affects general growth, particularly if corticosteroids have been given for long periods, even at low dosage around 3–5 mg of prednisolone daily.

Fractures

Fractures are not uncommon in children under five, especially if they have been immobilized for a long time. Crush fractures of vertebrae are largely confined to patients who have been treated with corticosteroids.

Amyloidosis

This is rare but usually proves fatal eventually. It is more common in patients with prolonged active disease, usually first manifesting itself with proteinuria, less often with anaemia or diarrhoea. It may progress to a nephrotic syndrome, uraemia and death, often proving fatal eight to ten years after its first appearance.

Death

Deaths in JCP are from amyloidosis with renal failure or from intercurrent infection. In Ansell's series infection was the most common single cause. Infective hepatitis, major liver necrosis and pancytopenia all play parts. Otherwise the prognosis in JCP is good, providing that joint function has been maintained and contractures avoided.

MANAGEMENT OF JCP

In all forms of juvenile polyarthritis, including juvenile rheumatoid arthritis and juvenile ankylosing spondylitis, the aims of treatment are to:

- Ease pain
- Suppress disease activity
- Prevent deformities
- Preserve function
- Maintain the child's education and normal mental and physical development.

The management is usually initiated in hospital but it must be continued at home and it is therefore important for the parents to play a central role from the start.

Prolonged bed rest is to be avoided unless absolutely necessary.

Physiotherapy and splintage, graded rest and exercises should be organized, with particular care to avoid flexion contractions which can occur insidiously but rapidly.

Joints may be splinted to prevent deformity: for example splints to be worn at night for wrists, knees and ankles; work splints for wrists and neck to be worn by day.

Skin traction may be used at night to overcome contraction of hips and knees. Hydrotherapy is popular and effective, and cycles and tricycles, first static, later mobile, are useful.

Nondrug management of JCP
- Avoid prolonged bed rest
- Physiotherapy
- Graded rest and exercise
- Splintage
- Skin traction
- Hydrotherapy

DRUG TREATMENT

The acute situation

NSAIDs   Aspirin is effective at a daily dose of 80 mg per kg body weight, as is aloxiprin at 130–150 mg 4-hourly for children of 3–6 years, 300–600 mg for ages 6–10 and 600–900 mg for 10–12-year olds, or 600 mg per 6.5 kg body weight daily in divided doses. Indomethacin 2.0 mg per kg per day in divided doses, ibuprofen 24–40 mg per kg per day, or tolmetin 20–30 mg per kg per day are alternatives. Indomethacin is not officially accepted for children in the United States but is found useful in Great Britain. (See also Chapter 29.)

Corticosteroids are useful to control acute episodes unresponsive to other measures, where general health is deteriorating, and in severe chronic iridocyclitis: prednisolone 10–20 mg by mouth as a single dose on alternate days, or corticotrophin by intramuscular (im) injection of 20 international units (iu) every 48 hours, or tetracosactrin by im injection of 0.1 mg every 2–3 days.

   These agents are easier to start than to stop and corticosteroid therapy should never be used unless it is absolutely necessary. When oral dosage is to be discontinued it should be reduced very gradually over a period of several weeks or even months. There are very real dangers associated with corticosteroid therapy in childhood. They include an increased risk of infection which may be fatal, retardation of growth, adrenocortical suppression, development of diabetes mellitus, cataract formation, moon face, Cushingoid obesity and other adverse reactions. (See also Chapter 30.)

Long-term agents

Antimalarials   For prolonged therapy chloroquine phosphate 4 mg per kg per day or hydroxychloroquine 5–7 mg per kg per day may be given. If no improvement has occurred after six months the drug should be discontinued but if there has been improvement at this time further dosage may be given on alternate days, the aim being to discontinue treatment after two years.

Corneal deposits of the drug may cause 'splintered vision' which disappears rapidly on reduction of dosage. However, as macular degeneration may occur – although rarely – initial and regular ocular checks are indicated.

Gold salts have been widely used. A suitable dose is 1 mg per kg of sodium aurothiomalate weekly, by im injection, ie, approximately 10 mg for children weighing up to 19 kg and 20 mg weekly for those weighing 20–30 kg.

Injections are given weekly for about six months, with close monitoring for proteinuria, blood dyscrasia or skin reactions. Blood and platelet counts must be done weekly at first, fortnightly later. Parents must test the urine weekly, using diagnostic 'sticks', and must report urinary abnormality or any rash as soon as it occurs.

If no benefit is seen after six months this treatment should be stopped but if there is improvement it should be continued for several months or years. When remission occurs, dosage should be reduced or given less frequently, at intervals of two, three or four weeks. It must be remembered that proteinuria may be a sign of amyloidosis rather than of gold intolerance.

D-penicillamine   The usefulness of this drug in childhood is still under assessment but comparisons with gold therapy seem to show that it is effective in oral doses of 50–100 mg daily, depending on whether the child's weight is under or over 20 kg. This dose may be increased if necessary by 50 mg a day at intervals of one or two months, with a maximum dosage of 450–600 mg, continuing for three years or so, depending on progress and toleration. The rules for monitoring of skin, urine, blood and platelets apply to d-penicillamine in the same way as for gold.

Immunosuppression   Azathioprine has been used at a dose of 2.5 mg per kg per day but is generally regarded as being too dangerous for routine use. Chlorambucil has been used to treat amyloidosis with doses of 0.15 mg per kg per day but monitoring is difficult and there are frequent complications, particularly the development of herpes zoster and chickenpox. These everyday infections are dangerous to the immuno-suppressed and often prove fatal.

Drug treatments for JCP

ACUTE SITUATION
- **NSAIDs**
  - aspirin
  - aloxiprin
  - indomethacin
  - ibuprofen
- **Corticosteroids**
  - prednisolone
  - corticotrophin
  - tetracosactrin

LONG-TERM
- **Antimalarials**
  - chloroquine phosphate
  - hydroxychloroquine
- **Gold salts**
  - sodium aurothiomalate
- **D-penicillamine**
- **Immunosuppressors**
  - azathioprine
  - chlorambucil

PROGNOSIS

Since the long-term prognosis in seronegative juvenile chronic polyarthritis is relatively good, it is as well not to be too heroic with potentially dangerous long-term therapy. Emphasis should be on control of pain, maintenance of function and avoidance of contractures. A good end result often comes as a pleasant surprise after years of active disease.

PRACTICAL POINTS

- JCP is a systemic disorder, with joints being one of the parts affected.
- There are two peak periods of age-incidence: at two to four and eleven to thirteen.
- Presentation may be as:
  —Systemic illness
  —Polyarthritis
  —Pauciarticular.
- Not all polyarticular disorders in children are JCP; there are many mimics.
- Management is based on the same principles as in adults: pain relief, anti-inflammatory drugs and graded exercises.
- Prognosis is often surprisingly good.

12
When is gout not gout?
Not even pseudogout?

Acute gout

One of the most characteristic clinical pictures is that of acute gout. When you ask a patient whether he has ever had gout and he answers 'What's that?' you can be certain he has never had an attack.

When an acute attack occurs in a usual place such as the big toe, which becomes very painful, red and tender, with desquamation over the joint as the attack abates, that is acute gout, whatever the circumstances and whatever the plasma uric acid level. If this level is high it does no more than help to confirm the diagnosis: acute gout occurs without hyperuricaemia and only a minority of people with hyperuricaemia develop acute gout.

Pseudogout

Other types of crystal deposition may cause similar syndromes – pseudogout – but usually in different areas.

Deposition of calcium pyrophosphate dihydrate (CPPD) in the tissues is most usually seen in the knees, less often in the hips, ankles, shoulders, elbows or wrists and very rarely in the great toe. CPPD deposition causes a low-grade arthritis resembling osteoarthrosis much more often than it causes acute pseudogout. The crystals are brick-shaped and weakly positively birefringent, readily distinguishable from urates.

Deposition of apatite crystals or injection of irritative corticosteroids may cause a similar inflammation, though rarely.

COMMON DIAGNOSTIC TRAPS

The big toe

1. Osteoarthrosis of a first metatarsophalangeal joint aggravated by trauma and often initiated by tight footwear may mimic acute gout quite closely, especially if there is inflammatory bursitis over the base of the toe with redness and swelling. As in gout the pain often follows exertion but it is only a modest ache when compared with gout which is usually agonizing and shows more florid signs of inflammation.

2. A March or other fracture may match gout for pain but there is no inflammatory reaction.

3. Cellulitis or other pyogenic infection may resemble gout and occasionally coexists with it when urate deposits and infection are both present and uratic material is found in the pus after drainage.

If both big toes are affected at the same time gout is unlikely. Gout is usually confined to one joint although if it is not rapidly controlled it may, if rarely, spread to or appear in another area.

True chronic gouty arthritis with tophi is rare in this country today and should become extinct now that uric acid levels can be held within the normal range and attacks can be prevented or rapidly controlled.

The ankle and foot

In the ankle or midtarsus the same considerations apply. A strain, dislocation or fracture may mislead but although pain and swelling are present heat and redness are minimal unless the part has been treated by warmth or local applications.

The knee

1. Pyarthrosis may resemble gout. Swelling, pain, heat, tenderness and redness are prominent. Constitutional disturbance is usually great and fever high.

2. Trauma or spontaneous fracture   The knee is seldom hot or red.

3. Rheumatoid and other arthritis   Pain is less severe. Heat and redness are less apparent.

4. Osteoarthrosis   Heat and redness are again less apparent. Effusion may be due to trauma, sometimes minor, or possibly to apatite crystal deposition.

When in doubt aspirate the effusion for cell counts, bacteriology and identification of crystals under the polarizing microscope.

The hand or wrist

In this area acute gout causes tense, hot, red or pink swelling of the tissues. Pyogenic infection may give a similar picture but fever and constitutional disturbance are likely to be greater.

Other joints

In the elbow, shoulder and other joints acute gout is very rare but its possibility must not be forgotten; however, gouty olecranon bursitis may occur.

Polyarticular gout is very rare indeed.

PRACTICAL POINTS IN DIAGNOSIS OF GOUT

There are certain features of a medical history which point towards a diagnosis of acute gout, whatever the site of the attack:

● **The patient has had such attacks in the past.** Familiarity does not, in this case, breed contempt. He usually makes his own diagnosis and is eager for early treatment.

● **Within the last twenty-four to thirty-six hours** the sufferer has had an acute illness or surgical operation, taken an effective diuretic, indulged in too much food, alcohol and/or exercise, or all three (eg, birthday, dinner-dance, wedding, football match and their consequent parties) or undergone a period of starvation and austerity (eg, crash diet, health farm). Any great break in the patient's routine seems likely to provoke an attack of gout and unwonted austerity seems to be as effective a trigger as unusual excess. For this reason gouty attacks often occur at weekends or on vacation or after long aeroplane flights. The wise patient always takes his favourite remedy in his hand baggage or pocket. Gout has a way of striking when pharmacies are shut and when bags that are not in the cabin have been misdirected *en route*.

● **The attack is more painful** than other joint episodes and the signs of inflammation are more marked.

● **The onset of pain** is often during the small hours, usually between 4 and 5 am.

13

Polymyalgia rheumatica: a forgotten syndrome

BACKGROUND

'Myalgic syndrome with constitutional effects: Polymyalgia rheumatica' was published by Stuart Barber in 1975.[1] The syndrome had already been described by several others who had given it names which implied that it was a form of rheumatoid arthritis occurring in old age or, in the case of one author, that it was a senile form of gout.

Barber had followed twelve sufferers from the syndrome for periods of up to ten years and found that none of them developed rheumatoid arthritis. He therefore insisted that this was a separate clinical entity and proposed the name of polymyalgia rheumatica. The great practical importance of his work was that it opened all our eyes to the fact that we each had several such cases under our care but were treating them as rheumatoid arthritis or osteoarthrosis and thereby denying them effective treatment.

DIAGNOSIS

Polymyalgia rheumatica can only be diagnosed after exclusion of other disorders, particularly rheumatoid arthritis and malignant disease. Its most important features are:

1. Painful morning stiffness of shoulder and pelvic girdles. The stiffness passes off in a few hours. Its dramatic response to corticosteroids in quite small doses suggests an inflammatory basis for the pain.
2. Very high erythrocyte sedimentation rate (ESR).
3. Rapid response to steroids.
4. Absence of joint involvement.
5. Absence of rheumatoid factor from the blood.
6. Absence of positive signs of other disorders.

ASSOCIATION WITH ARTERITIS

Polymyalgia rheumatica often appears to be a phase of giant cell-arteritis and the name of polymyalgia arteritica is preferred by some Scandinavian writers.[2] This may become the definitive name of the syndrome. In a seven-year survey of 75 patients in the south of England, A.B. Myles[3] found a simple polymyalgia picture in 52, cranial arteritis in 5 and a mixture in 18. Although joint symptoms and signs may be found in some cases and although some workers have found histological evidence of inflammation in joints, most rheumatologists now regard polymyalgia rheumatica as being due to inflammatory arteritis.

Arteritis is a common finding at biopsy and necropsy but there has been no evidence of primary myositis. In several reported cases treatment has been delayed pending biopsy of a painful artery, usually the temporal, and this has led to blindness from occlusion of a branch of the ophthalmic artery. Such delay can never be justified. A doctor who suspects arteritis should give at least 50 mg of prednisolone daily and arrange for biopsy as soon as possible.

COURSE AND OUTCOME

It is my experience that if patients diagnosed as suffering from polymyalgia rheumatica are followed up for several months they come to fall into one of three categories:

1. Those that improve within forty-eight hours, symptoms disappearing on doses of 15 mg of prednisolone or less daily, ESR falling, fever abating and the patient who has been considerably incapacitated being greatly improved, with improvement maintained during gradual reduction of the dose. In these cases the diagnosis was probably correct.
2. Those that show some improvement although it is less rapid, less complete and not so well maintained. The diagnosis remains possible, perhaps likely.
3. Those who show a poor response, initially and over the months. In these cases the diagnosis was probably wrong and we must look for another. When, we must ask ourselves, is 'polymyalgia rheumatica' not polymyalgia rheumatica?

WHAT ELSE MIGHT IT BE?

1. Rheumatoid arthritis?

In older people rheumatoid may take an acute polyarthritic form but it may start insidiously in shoulders and hips only. If other joints are involved, with swelling, pain and tenderness, the diagnosis will be obvious, but if rheumatoid factor is absent from the blood and if the arthritis is confined to hips and shoulders, rheumatoid may masquerade as polymyalgia rheumatica for several months with the response to steroid treatment being taken as confirmatory evidence.

I have seen three such patients, all over sixty-five, all of whom were misdiagnosed as polymyalgia rheumatica, the correct diagnosis becoming obvious in the subsequent six to twelve months.

2. Neoplastic (usually metastatic) disease?

Diffuse myalgia with a high ESR is quite common in malignant disease whether the primary growth is in the breast (the commonest site in women), the bronchus (the commonest site in men), the prostate, ovary, colon, thyroid or anywhere else. Patients with polymyalgia often have a febrile onset of their disease and they may lose weight at first, but if the weight loss progresses after the first month or two or if there are other features which suggest malignant disease, the diagnosis of polymyalgia rheumatica becomes less likely.

Hodgkin's disease and lymphoma seldom occur in this age group but multiple myeloma, with a median age occurrence at about sixty years, may cause acute bone and muscle pains with a raised ESR. It does not usually cause morning stiffness in the girdle areas.

3. A manifestation of chronic infection?

Tuberculosis of lungs, genito-urinary tract, bones, joints or alimentary canal, or even in the miliary form, may cause a similar syndrome, as may subacute bacterial endocarditis in the elderly. Abortus fever is now rare in this country and usually affects younger people. Salmonella infections can occur at any age and while most patients with acute disease are under middle age the chronic carrier state is more common after the age of fifty.

4. A manifestation of a disseminated connective tissue disease such as polymyositis or systemic lupus erythematosus?

These conditions usually occur at a younger age and have diagnostic changes in blood and electromyographs. Polymyositis usually presents insidiously as weakness in the proximal muscles of shoulder and hip.

MANAGEMENT

Control of polymyalgia rheumatica is with steroids. The Table right, above suggests dosage where there is no giant cell arteritis. The Table opposite is for cases of giant cell arteritis and should be followed in any case where eye involvement is suspected. Do not wait for a biopsy: one day's delay may lead to irreversible blindness. The doses may be varied for individual patients but if treatment is stopped or if dosage is lowered too rapidly there may be exacerbation and spread of symptoms.[4] Since the duration of the disease is often five to six years it is wise to continue treatment on the lowest effective dose for five to six years.

Complications

The only complications of treatment in Myles's[3] cases were crush fractures of vertebrae but I know of one woman who was receiving 9 mg of prednisolone daily and had excellent control of her polymyalgia when she contracted a fulminating pneumococcal infection and died of it.

Since polymyalgia rheumatica is a disease of old age many of its sufferers also have degenerative changes causing pain in neck, shoulders, hips and back. It is not always easy to decide which of the symptoms are due to polymyalgia and which are due to osteoarthrosis but if there is some pain which seems to be arthrotic it is sensible to add an NSAID such as indomethacin, ibuprofen, naproxen, fenbufen, indoprofen or piroxicam (see Chapter 29).

Guide to the treatment of polymyalgia rheumatica

1. Prednisolone 5 mg bd (but see 4).
2. When there is remission of symptoms and ESR is below 30 mm per hour reduce the daily dose by 0.5 mg every four weeks unless symptoms return or ESR rises. In which case:
3. Return to the previous dose for four weeks and then make a further attempt at reduction.
4. If adequate control is not achieved within five days on prednisolone 5 mg bd, increase to 5 mg tds. On remission reduce the daily dose by 1 mg every four weeks. When the daily dose is down to 10 mg, further reductions should be by 0.5 mg.
5. If adequate control is not achieved with 5 mg tds, reconsider the diagnosis.
6. If complete control is achieved, continue medication with normal sedimentation rate for up to a year before considering stopping treatment.

Guide to the treatment of giant cell arteritis

1. Start with prednisolone 20 mg daily (50–70 mg if there are ocular symptoms).
2. When control is achieved make weekly reductions of 2.5–5 mg daily.
3. When the dose is down to 20 mg a day make two-weekly reductions of 1 mg.
4. When the dose is down to 10 mg a day, make monthly reductions of 0.5 mg.
5. Continue treatment for up to a year with patient symptom free and sedimentation rate normal. Natural history of the disease may last several years. Treatment has therefore to be continued over this period in most cases.

WHAT PROGNOSIS?

Providing that the diagnosis is correct and the dosage of steroids adequate, then the condition should be completely controlled. The dosage of steroids will have to be decided by clinical trial, that is, the minimum dosage to control symptoms. Steroids will probably need to be taken for years. Again, clinical trial will be more helpful than ESR levels, though these are essential in assessing dose requirements.

There may be recurrences and patients will need to be told that they should report back or inform their physician by telephone on such occasions.

PRACTICAL POINTS

- Polymyalgia rheumatica is a disease that can be readily diagnosed and managed by the family doctor, if he is alert to it, confirms it with high ESR and prescribes steroids.
- Steroids are specific in controlling symptoms. If symptoms are not controlled the diagnosis is probably wrong.
- Steroids will be required for years, not months.
- Dosage will have to be tailored individually.

14
Disorders of bone

Disorders of bone may be local or generalized. They may be due to local specific disease or to systemic disorders in remote organs.

Clinical features of bone disorders may present as 'rheumatism' but practitioners must be alert to other possibilities.

OSTEOPOROSIS

This is a reduction in the amount of bone matrix (osteoid). There is a quantitative reduction in the amount of fully mineralized bone and this defect may lead to inability to withstand ordinary mechanical stresses and to provide adequate support. Calcium loss from bone is probably important. This thinning of the bone may be due to the following.

Causes

1. Disuse as when the patient remains inactive for a long period or when a bone is immobilized. Anyone who is crippled by arthritis or any other chronic disease is in danger of secondary osteoporosis. The risk increases with age.

2. Postmenopausal changes Oestrogen secretion diminishes at the menopause and osteoporosis, particularly of the spine, begins. It starts earlier if an artificial menopause has been induced.

In men osteoporosis begins in the late fifties or the sixties and is usually less marked than in women.

3. Old age Senile osteoporosis is partly due to androgen or oestrogen withdrawal, partly to disuse, and partly, in some cases, to deficient diet.

4. Hypogonadism as in eunuchoidism, Klinefelter's syndrome, ovarian agenesis and hypopituitarism.

5. Hyperthyroidism is a rare cause of osteoporosis which only occurs when severe disease has been present for some time without adequate treatment.

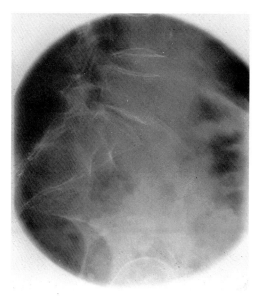

Figure 40 Osteoporosis of the lumbar spine in an elderly lady. The bone texture is thinned but no distortion has occurred (cf. crushed vertebra, Figure 79). The condition, apart from mild backache on occasion, is symptomless.

6. Adrenal cortical hyperfunction from Cushing's syndrome or prolonged treatment with corticosteroids.

7. Hyperparathyroidism may cause spinal osteoporosis, crush fractures, and softening and collapse of para-articular bone with reactive synovitis.

8. Inflammatory polyarthropathies including rheumatoid arthritis. There is osteoporosis in the area of the inflamed joints and this may be increased by disuse and possibly by corticosteroid treatment.

9. Dietary deficiency of protein and vitamin D is now rare in developed countries. Malabsorption with low calcium intake but adequate vitamin D may cause osteoporosis.

10. Diabetes mellitus Osteoporosis may occur but is seldom a problem.

Biochemistry

In osteoporosis not secondary to endocrine disorders serum calcium is either normal or slightly lowered, and serum alkaline phosphatase and phosphate levels are normal.

Treatment

Rest is necessary for acute pain that may be caused by crush fractures of porotic vertebrae, and the spine must be supported in a good anatomical position. But prolonged rest will aggravate the porosis and there must therefore be graded mobilization as soon as the acute symptoms have abated with the help of adequate analgesia (see Chapter 32).

Calcium supplements (calcium lactate 300 mg tds – or more, up to 5 g daily – or calcium gluconate 600 mg three to six times a day) will help to correct any deficiency. Microcrystalline calcium hydroxyapatite (MCHC) as a powder or tablets (up to 3 g daily, in divided doses taken before meals) is a useful preparation that provides calcium and phosphorus in a protein base. Vitamin D (1,000–1,500 iu daily by mouth) will help calcium absorption but larger doses may cause renal stones.

Oestrogens are said to prevent or improve menopausal osteoporosis. Ethinyl oestradiol (0.2 mg) or conjugated equine oestrogens in graded dosage given daily for three weeks in each month appear to prevent bone loss and improve the absorption of calcium, but the monthly withdrawal bleeding is sometimes unpleasantly profuse and there are still doubts as to whether long-term treatment of this kind may carry an increased risk of uterine carcinoma. Beneficial effects also may wear off after around one to two years.

The treatment of osteoporosis is by no means simple unless there is a primary cause such as thyrotoxicosis or Cushing's syndrome, which can be ascertained and corrected. Otherwise it is rest followed by mobilization with calcium supplements and perhaps conservative doses of vitamin D, and possibly oestrogens in selected cases.

OSTEOMALACIA

Osteomalacia is due to defective calcification of osteoid.

Causes

1. **Rickets**, rare in children, not so rare in geriatric practice.
2. **Malabsorption** as after partial gastrectomy.
3. **Chronic renal failure**: 'renal rickets' with hypocalcaemia, hyperphosphataemia and metabolic acidosis. Phosphate-losing renal disease may also cause osteomalacia: serum calcium and phosphorus concentrations are usually low but in hypophosphataemia calcium levels are usually normal.
4. **Secondary hyperparathyroidism** may occur, especially in renal disease and with hypocalcaemic patients.

Symptoms

These include pains in the lower limbs and the spine where they often seem to be muscular rather than spinal. More acute pains suggest crush or stress fracture. Bony

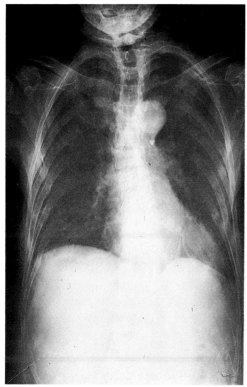

Figure 41   Gross osteomalacia in an elderly lady with marked deformation of the thoracic cage and fractures of ribs.

tenderness may be marked. There may be pain in the region of the hips and a waddling gait. With low levels of serum calcium muscular weakness, hypotonia and – rarely – tetany may occur.

Treatment

Treatment is, if possible, directed at the cause.

For vitamin D deficiency give calciferol up to 2,000–4,000 iu daily with calcium supplement.

Renal osteomalacia may be resistant and need 100,000 iu daily but serum calcium must be carefully monitored.

In glomerular failure renal tubular acidosis must be corrected with bicarbonate, electrolytes and glucose for hypoglycaemia.

In renal tubular failure phosphate supplements (1 g daily) are needed.

In steatorrhoea a gluten-free diet may restore the calcium balance to normal. The diet must always be studied and improved as necessary, particularly in the case of postgastrectomy patients.

OSTEITIS FIBROSA CYSTICA

Causes

Osteitis fibrosa cystica is due to primary or secondary hyperparathyroidism, which causes resorption of minerals from the bones.

The primary form is due to an excessive secretion of parathormone due to parathyroid hyperplasia or an adenoma. Excess of parathormone affects:

1. The bones, to cause hydroxyapatite breakdown with release of calcium.
2. The renal tubules, to cause increased phosphorus excretion.

The secondary form is due to renal disease.

Symptoms

Serum calcium is raised as is the alkaline phosphatase when there is new bone formation. The serum phosphorus is low except in renal failure when it rises. A twenty-four hour specimen of urine will show increased amounts of calcium and phosphorus. General bone pains and tenderness are common. There may be nausea, vomiting and muscle weakness. Band keratitis (corneal calcification), peptic ulceration, pancreatitis and renal calcification may be present in some cases. X-rays show diffuse osteoporosis with bone cysts.

Treatment

Treatment is that of the primary condition: eg, parathyroidectomy for primary hyperparathyroidism.

PAGET'S DISEASE OF BONE (OSTEITIS DEFORMANS)

Although there may be periods of pain lasting weeks or months, Paget's disease is usually symptomless and discovered by chance when X-rays reveal typical patchy bone density against less dense and sometimes cystic areas. Around 1 per cent of people over the age of forty-five are said to have these X-ray changes somewhere in their bodies but only a minority have symptoms. The serum alkaline phosphatase is raised.

This disease is characterized by bone absorption and concurrent new bone formation, the cause of which is unknown. The new bone is poor in calcium but rich in blood vessels, with many arteriovenous shunts.

Symptoms

Paget's disease may become evident clinically when the cranium has enlarged so that the patient finds his hat to be fitting more tightly, with his forehead bulging forward.

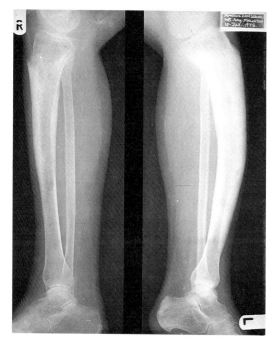

Figure 42   Paget's disease of tibiae in
an elderly lady. Changes are slight on
the right but with marked bowing and
bone thickening on the left.

Deafness is common. Diabetes insipidus may result from compression of the pituitary
but this is rare. Long bones may become thickened, bent and warmer to the touch. Any
long bone may be affected, but the bent and thickened 'sabre' tibia is the most obvious.
The spine is often involved. There is usually nothing to be seen on examination of the
spine but kyphosis increases gradually and acute painful episodes may be caused by
crush fractures or by small bony cracks which are not visible in X-rays. Fractures often
occur without back pain or tenderness and without pain on movement. Sarcomatous
changes occur in a very few cases.

Biochemistry

The serum alkaline phosphatase is raised in Paget's disease but calcium and phosphorus
are normal. Urinary hydroxyproline is increased as a result of osteoclastic activity.

Treatment

Analgesics for acute painful episodes are usually all that is needed but calcitonin
inhibits bone resorption and will relieve pain eventually. It may be given by
subcutaneous injection in 30 doses of 160 units either daily or on alternate days. Local
radiotherapy may relieve pain.

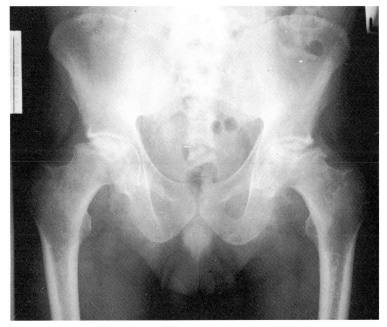

Figure 43 Avascular necrosis of hips.

AVASCULAR ASEPTIC BONE NECROSIS

This follows infarction due to interference with local blood supply. It affects the hips most commonly.

Necrosis confined to one area may follow injury, rheumatoid disease or osteoarthrosis, but it may be impossible to determine the cause.

More widespread necrosis affecting hips and shoulders may occur in caisson (decompression) disease of professional divers, in diabetes mellitus, sickle cell disease, chronic alcoholism, systemic lupus erythematosus or pancreatitis and it may occur as a complication of prolonged treatment with large doses of corticosteroids.

Treatment

Treatment is usually conservative with analgesics, physiotherapy and attention to the underlying disease, but hip replacement is sometimes needed.

MALIGNANT DISEASE

Sarcomas

Paget's sarcoma has already been mentioned in this chapter, and other forms of sarcoma may be found.

Metastatic deposits from distant primary sites seldom affect joints but secondary deposits may occur in bone, particularly from carcinoma of lung, breast, prostate, kidney, thyroid and gastro-intestinal tract. Such secondaries are usually osteolytic, causing pain and pathological fractures. Osteosclerotic deposits are usually secondary to carcinoma of the prostate.

Multiple myeloma

This is probably the most common bone neoplasm. It may be widely disseminated in the skeleton causing fractures and painful periosteal reactions in the long bones and crush fractures of the spine. Patients are usually over the age of forty. Multiple myeloma is a highly malignant plasma cell tumour of the bone marrow and is characterized by overproduction of IgG, IgA, IgD or IgE. There is a high ESR with anaemia, and a myeloma band in the electrophoretic strip. Bence-Jones protein may be found in the urine, and serum calcium may be raised. X-rays show lytic lesions, often multiple.

Treatment

Chemotherapy with melphalan or cyclophosphamide is often necessary. Other treatment is with local radiotherapy and analgesics as required. Corticosteroids may be necessary if hypercalcaemia is present, with allopurinol to control the hyperuricaemia which may be dangerous to the kidney. Amputation may have to be considered in the case of primary tumours of bone.

Hodgkin's disease

In this condition bone involvement may produce pain and rarefaction, vertebral compression and, rarely, fractures. Diagnosis is by biopsy of an accessible lesion and treatment by chemotherapy and/or radiation.

Finally, note that primary malignant disease of bone may occur in young people, and the diagnosis missed unless the possibility is considered.

OSTEOMYELITIS

Osteomyelitis is now uncommon but must be remembered as a possibility in any bone lesion. Acute haematogenous osteomyelitis is due to S. Aureus in 80 per cent of cases and must be treated by early administration of the appropriate antibiotic; preceded by blood culture, biopsy or swab to determine the causative bacteriological organism. The antibiotic should be administered for eight to twelve weeks after all swelling and tenderness have subsided and the bone must be immobilized by plaster or traction until all signs of active infection have settled. A local abscess needs surgical drainage. Delay leads to a chronic bone abscess with destructive changes; all dead and infected bone then has to be removed.

PRACTICAL POINTS

● **Osteoporosis** Longer life-expectancy means that the number of people suffering from osteoporosis is growing. A painful disorder, difficult to control.

● **Osteomalacia** A rare disorder, secondary to some general conditions such as deficiency of vitamin D and chronic renal failure.

● **Osteitis fibrosa cystica** is due to hyperparathyroidism.

● **Paget's disease of bone** is very prevalent in elderly. It is often symptomless.

● **Avascular aseptic necrosis** causes damage to bones, especially in hips and shoulders.

● **Malignant diseases** may be secondary or primary, and require clinical alertness for diagnosis.

● **Osteomyelitis**, though rare, should be considered in a sick febrile patient with a painful joint or limb.

15
Compression neuropathies

BACKGROUND

Pain due to compression or entrapment of a nerve is often first thought to be due to some form of arthritis. The most common features of compression or entrapment are:

1. Pain, worse at night, with abnormal sensations in the distribution of the compressed nerve.
2. Pain may be felt above and below the site of compression but paraesthesiae are only felt below the compression.
3. At first there are only symptoms. Physical signs appear later.

The more common compression syndromes are listed in the Table below.

The commoner compression syndromes
- **Upper limb**
  - Carpal tunnel syndrome
  - Ulnar tunnel syndrome
  - Ulnar nerve compression at the elbow
  - Pronator syndrome
  - Posterior interosseous nerve compression
  - Anterior interosseous nerve syndrome
  - Dorsal scapular nerve compression
- **Lower limb**
  - Tarsal tunnel syndrome
  - Peroneal nerve compression
  - Meralgia paraesthetica
  - Ilio-inguinal nerve compression
  - Obturator nerve compression
  - Sciatic nerve compression
  - Saphenous nerve compression
  - Nerve compression in the foot (Morton's metatarsalgia)

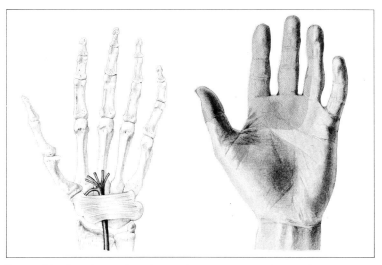

Figure 44 Carpal tunnel syndrome showing sensory changes from median nerve compression at wrist.

CARPAL TUNNEL SYNDROME

This is the most common of the compression syndromes. It occurs frequently in rheumatoid arthritis and may be the first manifestation of that disease. It may also occur in pregnancy, acromegaly, myxoedema, multiple myeloma or amyloidosis, or after an injury to the wrist such as a Colles' fracture. Usually there are no underlying causes found.

The median nerve is compressed in the carpal tunnel causing pain in the wrist and hand which often radiates up the arm, particularly at night when the patient experiences numbness, tingling and other odd sensations in the arm and in the lateral three and a half fingers of the hand, sparing the ulnar nerve distribution (see diagram above).

Carpal tunnel syndrome most often occurs as an idiopathic entity, apparently not secondary to any other condition. In such cases it is most common in women over forty and generally affects the dominant hand. In rare bilateral cases the dominant hand is usually the worse. This condition may be due to hard work which involves compression of the hand and wrist against a hard surface, as in scrubbing or ironing.

Compression of the median nerve may cause wasting of the muscles of the thenar eminence. There may be cutaneous sensory loss over the thumb and index, middle and radial half of ring fingers. Abduction and apposition of the thumb may be impaired. Numbness and paraesthesiae of the lateral three and a half digits precede muscle weakness and atrophy. Percussion of the nerve on the palmar aspect of the wrist may cause paraesthesiae (Tinel's sign). Flexion of the hand at the wrist for over a minute

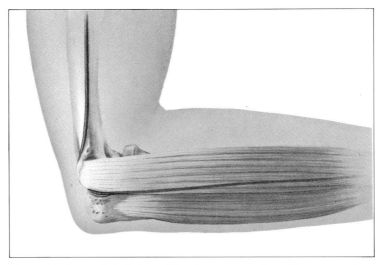

Figure 45 Anatomical relations of the ulnar nerve at elbow. The nerve reaches a groove behind the medial epicondyle then passes down the forearm between flexor carpi ulnaris and flexor digitorum profundus muscles.

Figure 46 Ulnar nerve distribution of sensory change with ulnar nerve compression at elbow.

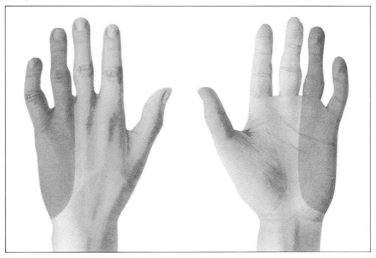

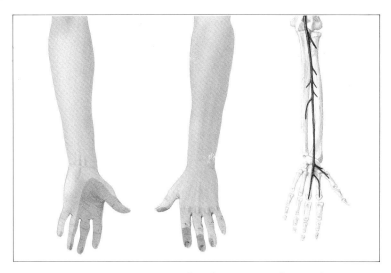

Figure 47 Pronator compression of median nerve at elbow with sensory changes.

(Phalen's manoeuvre) usually produces pain and paraesthesiae. There may be minimal or no physical signs in mild cases.

When carpal tunnel syndrome is the first sign of rheumatoid arthritis there is usually some morning stiffness of the fingers with tenderness of the metacarpal heads and slight tenderness and swelling of the proximal interphalangeal joints as well as tenderness around the wrist itself.

Treatment

In most cases it is best to play for time. If the condition is not severe it may subside spontaneously. A local steroid injection is often helpful (see Chapter 31). In other cases the application of a splint will enable the condition to settle down within a few weeks, but it is often necessary to release the nerve by dividing the flexor retinaculum.

ULNAR TUNNEL COMPRESSION

The ulnar nerve may be compressed at the wrist, causing pain and paraesthesiae on the ulnar side of the hand and impairment of sensation in the medial one and a half fingers. There may be some wasting of the small muscles of the hand. If the deep branch of the nerve is involved, some wasting is noted but there is no sensory loss. This may be due to pressure by a ganglion, injury, or – rarely – rheumatoid arthritis or long-distance cycling.

Treatment

Treatment is by excision of the volar carpal ligament or ganglion.

ULNAR NERVE COMPRESSION AT THE ELBOW

This is usually caused by the fibrous arch of origin of flexor carpi ulnaris but it may follow a condylar fracture or be due to a ganglion, arthritis of the elbow or an unusually mobile ulnar nerve.

There is pain in the hand with impaired sensation in the medial one and a half fingers and the palm, sometimes with wasting of the small muscles. There may also be pain in the forearm.

Treatment

Division of the fibrous arch is usually sufficient but it is sometimes necessary to transplant the ulnar nerve. Elbow synovectomy may be required if due to severe rheumatoid arthritis.

Entrapment of ulnar nerve

At the wrist	At the elbow
1. Normal motor function flexor carpi ulnaris and flexor digitorum profundus and intrinsic muscles of 4th and 5th digits.	1. Weakness flexor carpi ulnaris and flexor digitorum profundus and intrinsic muscles of 4th and 5th digits.
2. Sensory loss on palm only, not on dorsum of hand.	2. Sensory loss extends to dorsum of ulnar side of hand.
3. Electrodiagnostic testing shows delayed motor and sensory terminal latencies of ulnar nerve in the hand.	3. Electrodiagnosis localizes the area of entrapment.

Both median and ulnar nerves may also become entrapped in the lower cervical spine from spondylosis C8-T1, or in the thoracic inlet giving rise to the 'double crush' syndrome with both nerves affected. X-rays of the neck and electrodiagnostic tests are necessary for correct diagnosis.

PRONATOR SYNDROME

This is caused by compression of the median nerve by the pronator teres or the fibrous arch of origin of flexor digitorum sublimis. Symptoms are similar to those of the carpal tunnel syndrome (see page 113). Conduction studies show delay at forearm level.

This syndrome affects the dominant hand. Symptoms may be worse after hard work, particularly if it involves repetitive movements of pronation. They are not worse at night.

Treatment

The nerve must be decompressed.

POSTERIOR INTEROSSEOUS NERVE COMPRESSION

The posterior interosseous nerve is purely a motor branch of the radial nerve. Compression occurs at the fibrous origin of extensor carpi radialis brevis or between the two heads of supinator. There is pain over the lateral epicondyle of the elbow and tenderness around the extensor origin. Symptoms are identical with those of 'tennis elbow' and an alternative diagnosis of interosseous compression must be considered if a case of 'tennis elbow' does not respond to treatment.

Treatment

If the nerve has not been divided by pressure or injury recovery will take place within eight to twelve weeks. Steroid injections into the elbow may help if compression is due to rheumatoid arthritis (see Chapter 10). In resistant cases synovectomy and decompression, or tendon transfer may be necessary.

ANTERIOR INTEROSSEOUS NERVE SYNDROME

This is due to the compression of this nerve, a purely motor branch of the median, by the pronator quadratus, flexor pollicis longus and flexor digitorum profundus of the index and middle fingers. The patient often complains of pain in the forearm and elbow and has weakness in the above muscles of these two digits or sometimes only of the flexor pollicis or the flexor digitorum profundus of the index fingers.

Treatment

Spontaneous recovery may occur in six weeks to six months or may take up to eighteen months. Surgical decompression of the nerve may be necessary.

DORSAL SCAPULAR NERVE COMPRESSION

The dorsal scapular nerve may be compressed by the scalenus medius muscle which it runs through to serve the rhomboid muscles that hold and stabilize the scapula against the chest wall. It has no skin sensory distribution. Weakness and atrophy of these muscles may lead to winging of the scapula on wide abduction of the arm, and aching is most marked along the medial border of the scapula, diffusing less severely over the lateral surface of arm and forearm. It may follow a little time after violent head jarring. The head is held stiffly tilted away from the affected side and flexion and rotation to that side increases the pain and increases radiation into the arm. There may be puffiness in the supraclavicular area. The rhomboids are tender as are the lower two-thirds of the scalenus medius, pressure causing pain locally and radiating down into the forearm.

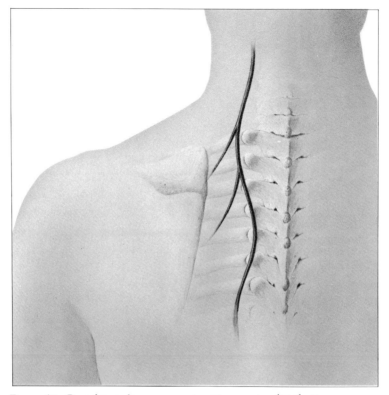

Figure 48   Dorsal scapular nerve compression: motor distribution.

Treatment

Treatment is to immobilize with a collar, to give analgesics, sedation and physiotherapy. Traction may sometimes help. If the scalenus muscle is divided care must be taken to avoid the nerve.

TARSAL TUNNEL SYNDROME

This results from compression of the posterior tibial nerve by the lancinate ligament which roofs the tarsal tunnel between the medial malleolus and the os calcis.

There is burning pain with paraesthesiae in the toes and sole, worse at night and usually relieved by hanging the limb out of bed or by movement. The pain may radiate up the leg in the sciatic distribution and can be mistaken for sciatica. Sensory loss may be confined to the medial three and a half toes and the sole, or to the lateral one and a half toes and the sole, or sometimes to the heel only, depending on the branch affected.

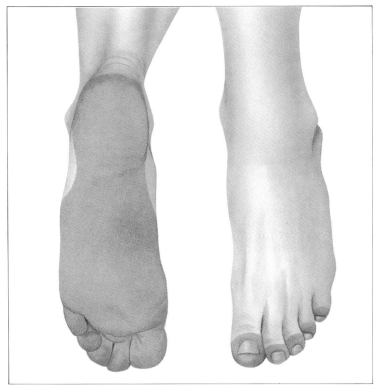

Figure 49   Sensory distribution affected by tarsal tunnel compression of the posterior tibial nerve behind and below the medial malleolus.

Treatment

Local steroid injection may help. Surgical decompression is sometimes necessary.

PERONEAL COMPRESSION

This occurs as the nerve winds round the neck of the fibula. It may be caused by a tight plaster or boot, or by direct injury. Pain is felt at the lateral side of the leg and foot. There may be sensory change over the distal lateral aspect of the leg and the dorsum of the foot, and muscular weakness may cause what the patient describes as 'a weak ankle', the foot tending to become inverted on walking. Eversion of the foot and dorsiflexion at ankles and toes are all weakened.

Treatment

A lateral wedge on the sole helps to maintain eversion. Surgery is sometimes needed to free and decompress the nerve by detaching a small portion of peroneus longus.

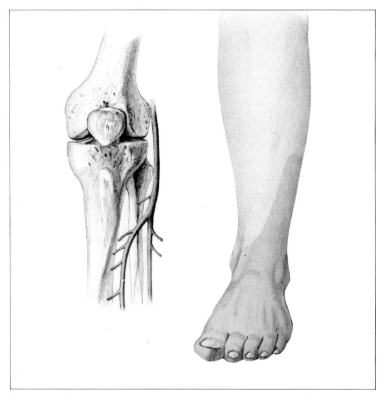

Figure 50   Common peroneal nerve compression with area of sensory involvement.

MERALGIA PARAESTHETICA

There is burning pain with numbness, paraesthesia and hyperalgaesia over the lateral part of the thigh. Symptoms and signs are entirely sensory. There is no motor weakness. This syndrome is thought to be due to compression of the lateral femoral cutaneous nerve at the anterior superior iliac spine where it passes to the lateral end of the inguinal ligament, or where it pierces the iliac fascia. But it is similar to the 'right-about-turn syndrome', so called because sometimes the infantryman causes root injury in his lumbar spine when he swings his body smartly round and stamps his foot on the hard parade ground.

Treatment

Local injection of prednisolone is often helpful. An operation is seldom needed.

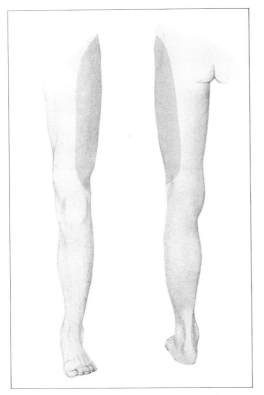

Figure 51   Area of hypoaesthesia in meralgia paraesthetica due to lateral femoral cutaneous nerve compression.

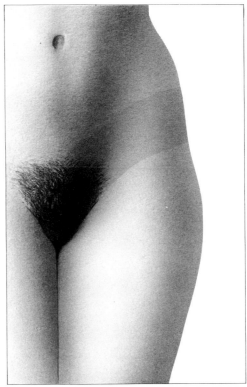

Figure 52   Ilio-ilingual nerve sensory distribution.

ILIO-INGUINAL AND OBTURATOR NERVE COMPRESSIONS

These cause pain in the groin which may be mistaken for hip pain. The syndrome may be caused by bursae pressing on the nerve. There is sensory loss below the inguinal ligament and on the inner side of the thigh. Symptoms are aggravated by standing or excessive hip movements. The patient may walk bent forward to relieve the pain and may sleep with the thigh flexed. Hyperaesthesia may be marked, with a point of maximal tenderness on pressure just above the anterior superior iliac spine. Pain is aggravated by extending the hip and contracting the lower abdominal muscles.

Treatment

Injection of local anaesthetic and/or corticosteroid solution may help. Surgical decompression is sometimes needed.

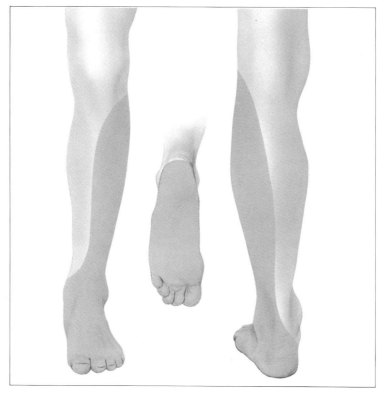

Figure 53   Sensory distribution of sciatic nerve compression.

SCIATIC NERVE COMPRESSION

This may have many causes but true entrapment of the nerve itself is comparatively rare. More common are: root compression or irritation by a prolapsed intervertebral disc, a growth, or an inflammation. Pressure on the sciatic nerve during its course may be due to a hip prosthesis or to the piriformis muscle trapping the nerve at the greater sciatic notch (the piriformis syndrome) with motor and sensory signs distal to the lesion and closely resembling a lumbar disc syndrome. Prolonged squatting may nip the nerve as it runs between the ischial tuberosity and the great trochanter, or where it reaches the thigh between adductor magnus and the hamstrings. The sciatic nerve may be compressed behind the knee by a Baker's cyst (semimembranosus bursa) in a patient with rheumatoid arthritis.

In sciatic nerve compression from a neoplasm the onset is gradual and the symptoms are progressive, with muscle wasting more apparent and sensory loss greater.

Sciatic nerve compression is often wrongly diagnosed, any pain that radiates down the leg being attributed to sciatic compression.

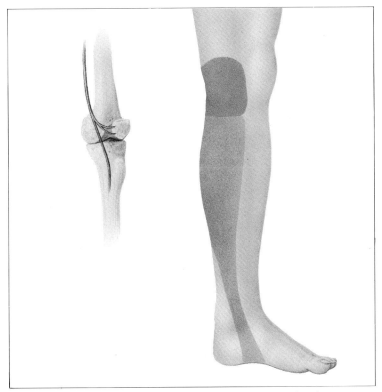

Figure 54 Saphenous nerve branch of the femoral nerve distribution to the leg.

Treatment

This depends on the cause. In most cases conservative treatment with rest and analgesics is all that is necessary. In a few cases of the piriformis syndrome it is necessary to expose the nerve surgically and free it from compression.

SAPHENOUS NERVE COMPRESSION

This occurs at the lower end of the adductor (Hunter's) canal where the nerve pierces the aponeurotic roof of the canal. There is pain on the medial side of the knee, radiating down the medial aspect of the leg to the inner side of the foot and big toe. Friction against the posterior border of the sartorius muscle during limb movements may simulate the pain of intermittent claudication.

Treatment

Injections of local anaesthetic at the point of maximum tenderness is often effective. It may have to be repeated. Surgical decompression is sometimes necessary.

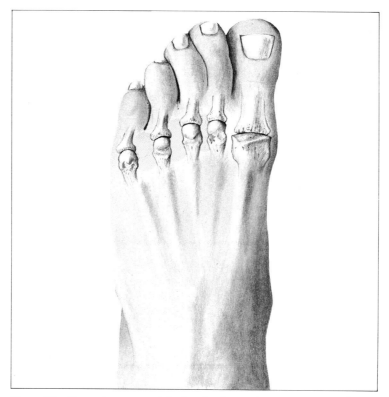

Figure 55   Morton's metatarsalgia showing bursae between metatarsal heads of 2–5 digits.

MORTON'S METATARSALGIA

Nerve compression in the foot occurs from pressure on the plantar digital nerves by the metatarsal heads and the small bursae which lie between them. This occurs most commonly between the heads of the third and fourth metatarsals; there is no bursa between the heads of the first and second. Repeated compression may cause fibrosis or a neuroma.

Symptoms vary. Sharp stabbing pains in the region of the metatarsal heads, radiating into the toes, occur initially on walking but later also during rest at night. In the day the patient will slip off his shoe and rub the foot to get relief. The pain may be throbbing and its distribution depends on the nerve affected. The lesion is most often between the third and fourth metatarsal heads, less often between the second and third. There may be swelling and tenderness between the metatarsal heads and there is sometimes diminished sensation between the affected toes.

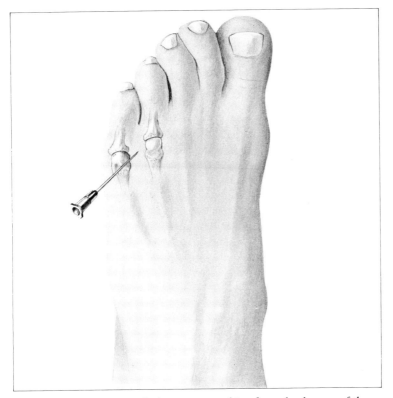

Figure 56   Injecting into the bursa, approaching from the dorsum of the foot.

Treatment

Symptoms are often relieved by injection of lignocaine into the bursae which should be approached from the dorsum of the foot. A painful neuroma must be excised.

PRACTICAL POINTS

● In many compression neuropathies radiographs and electrodiagnostic studies are necessary before a correct diagnosis can be made.
● Compression may exert its harmful effect by mechanical pressure or distortion of the nerve or, sometimes, by inducing ischaemic changes in it.

16

Some unusual arthropathies

BACKGROUND

Although by definition these arthropathies are rare in practice, probably occurring once in a professional lifetime, they are of particular interest and serve as challenges in diagnosis and management.

There are well over 100 disorders of bone and joint and although some twelve conditions cover the large majority of cases other more unusual conditions turn up from time to time. I have seen the following recently.

THE ARTHROPATHIES

Sarcoidosis

A man of twenty-five had walked fairly briskly round one of the larger London parks a month previously. On rising next day he found that he had difficulty in walking because his ankles and knees were stiff. The stiffness improved after simple activity but became worse again after each night's rest.

Two weeks previously the patient had had a sore throat with 'flu-like' symptoms. This was followed by swelling of the ankles and red, raised patches over the shins (erythema nodosum). His doctor had already made the diagnosis of sarcoid arthropathy and brought his X-ray, which showed typical hilar gland enlargement. The ankles were tender and swollen but the knees and hands, which had been affected, had settled. The patient's temperature was 37.5°C; his pulse, 84.

Erythema nodosum and the typical X-ray were the diagnostic pointers. Before 1939 erythema nodosum was usually a reaction to infection with haemolytic streptococci or the tubercle bacillus, but since then the commonest cause in developed countries has been sarcoidosis. The rash, usually confined to the front of the shins, is raised, tender, red and initially painful. The lesions, about 6 mm in diameter, are circular or irregular in shape with normal surrounding skin. The arthropathy may take either of two forms.

1. **Early, acute and transient** with erythema nodosum in 70 per cent of cases and polyarthritis in 40–50 per cent, both occurring at or soon after the first onset of

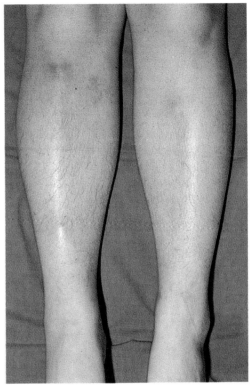

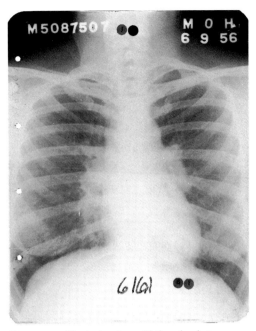

Figure 58   Typical enlarged hilar glands in sarcoidosis.

Figure 57   Erythema nodosum over the front of the shin of the right leg. Such lesions are usually multiple.

symptoms, as in the case just described. The arthritis is usually symmetrical, affecting knees and ankles most often but also, on occasion, elbows, wrists, shoulders and the metacarpophalangeal and proximal interphalangeal joints of the hands. The skin lesions last up to six months and may recur. The arthritis usually subsides completely within six months.

The intracutaneous tuberculin test (Mantoux) is negative. The Kveim test (a granulomatous reaction appearing four weeks after intradermal injection of sarcoid material) is usually but not invariably positive. The ESR is raised. It is, however, as well to remember that primary tuberculosis, streptococcal infection, drug sensitivity (eg, to sulphonamide), leprosy, ulcerative colitis and Crohn's disease, as well as some other conditions, including malignant growth, are occasionally associated with erythema nodosum.

Treatment is by rest, graded activity and an NSAID (see Chapters 29 and 32).

2. The chronic persistent type of polyarthritis associated with chronic sarcoidosis in about 10 per cent of cases, is most common (3:1) in women, usually between the ages of fifteen and thirty. The arthritis has the distribution described above and is usually symmetrical. Rarely it affects the big toe to resemble gout. Other manifestations are peripheral lymphadenopathy (80 per cent), cutaneous sarcoid (50 per cent) and iritis (30 per cent). Radiographs show hilar lymphadenopathy in most cases and lung infiltration in 50 per cent. This condition lasts for years with remissions but usually subsides completely with few or no permanent changes.

Treatment is with NSAIDs and analgesics. Corticosteroids are only needed for severe cases that refuse to respond and for patients with severe iritis or hypercalcaemia (see Chapters 29 and 30).

Palindromic rheumatism

This arthropathy was first described and named by Hench and Rosenberg in the American forces (1944). They described recurrent acute self-limited attacks of arthritis lasting only a few days or sometimes only a few hours, with pain, stiffness and swelling of hands, wrists, feet and knees most commonly; of shoulders, elbows and ankles quite often; and of hips and jaws occasionally. There is complete recovery from each attack. The attacks may occur every few weeks, the average frequency being twenty a year, but they may occur more frequently or disappear for a few years.

Hench and Rosenberg thought this syndrome to be an individual entity but I have seen several patients become typical cases of rheumatoid arthritis and others who proved to be cases of systemic lupus erythematosus. Many cases (about half) continue for years and then subside. It is likely that in most cases in Great Britain the underlying condition is rheumatoid arthritis of a mild and relapsing nature.

Treatment is symptomatic but there is some evidence that 250 mg of d-penicillamine taken daily, or injections of gold salts weekly or fortnightly, will prevent relapses.

Pseudohypertrophic pulmonary osteoarthropathy

The patient, usually a man, presents with loss of weight, failing health and swelling and discomfort in joints, usually in knees, ankles and feet although arm joints may also be affected. Pain is rarely severe. The essential diagnostic sign is clubbing of the fingers. Although there are many causative conditions, as listed in the Table opposite, the commonest cause is carcinoma, usually of the bronchus, usually peripheral and subpleural. Primary tumours of pleura, mediastinum, diaphragm and upper gastro-intestinal tract may also be responsible, although less frequently.

This arthropathy appears early in cases of malignant disease but in others it may only

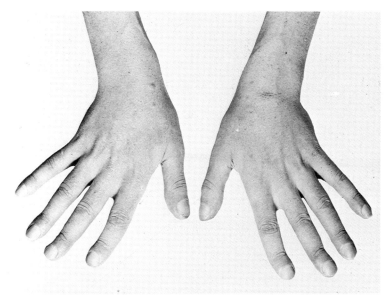

Figure 59 Clubbing of fingers in pseudohypertrophic pulmonary osteoarthropathy due to a bronchial carcinoma.

appear years after the onset of the primary condition. Thickening of extremities and occasionally of features may suggest acromegaly.

X-rays show periosteal elevation of the shafts of long bones of forearms, hands and legs below the knee. Aspiration of fluid from affected joints reveals a noninflammatory picture, white cells being fewer than 2,000 per cu mm, mostly mononuclears.

Treatment is palliative but removal of the malignant growth may lead to rapid resolution or improvement in the arthritic condition, as may ligature of a major vessel to the growth or a vagotomy.

Causes of pseudohypertrophic pulmonary osteoarthropathy

1. Malignant and benign primary and secondary tumours of lung, pleura, heart, diaphragm, mediastinum or upper gastro-intestinal tract.
2. Pulmonary suppuration (empyema, lung abscess, emphysema, bronchiectasis).
3. Gastro-intestinal disorders (ulcerative colitis, Crohn's disease, steatorrhoea, hepatic cirrhosis).
4. Cyanotic congenital heart disease.
5. Aortic aneurysm (the clubbing may be unilateral).

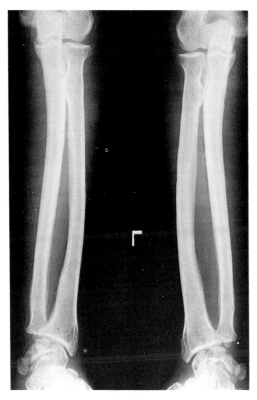

Figure 60 Periosteal elevation of bones of forearms in the same patient.

The knuckle-pad syndrome

Also known as Garrod's fatty pads or as Hale-White's nodes, this is an indolent condition of no pathological but considerable diagnostic importance which may be confused with more serious conditions such as rheumatoid arthritis. I see about four new cases every year. The patient, male or female and of any age, notices fleshy pads 2–3 mm in diameter over the dorsum of the proximal interphalangeal joints of the fingers. They are usually symptomless. Pain and tenderness are unusual but add to the diagnostic confusion if they occur. The pads are fibrofatty and are not inflamed. This condition may be associated with Dupuytren's contracture and it may be hereditary.

Treatment The patient can be reassured that he has not got arthritis. No other treatment is necessary. Some women patients think the lesions are unsightly and wish to have them removed but in most cases they are only noticed by the patient herself.

Teitze's syndrome

This is another condition of no serious importance for which the best treatment is reassurance. The patient, of any age and either sex, notices painful swelling of a costal cartilage, usually the second or third, sometimes the first or fourth, usually at the costosternal junction, usually at only one site. Where more than one site is affected the disorder is unilateral in 80 per cent of cases.

The patient complains that the cartilage is painful, tender and swollen, the pain being aggravated by coughing or sneezing. There is no history of injury or strain. There is nothing to be found on examination apart from tenderness over a prominent costal cartilage. All investigations, including biopsy, are negative. The condition may come on rapidly or slowly, the pain lasting for some hours or several days, recurring at irregular intervals and usually disappearing for ever within a year.

The differential diagnosis must exclude inflammatory disease (pyogenic and tuberculous) of the chest wall, ankylosing spondylitis, leukaemia, disease of heart, lung, pericardium and pleura and malignancy. This is an odd disorder whose origin remains quite unexplained. In my own experience of patients who presented in this way I have usually found no disease process, but ankylosing spondylitis and leukaemia can both cause chest pain and I have seen two cases of infection, one due to tuberculosis, the other to low-grade paratyphoid fever.

Treatment is symptomatic following adequate investigation and firm reassurance.

Ochronosis (alkaptonuria)

This is a rare hereditary disease in which deficiency of the enzyme homogentisic acid oxidase is transmitted as an autosomal recessive character.

Homogentisic acid is excreted in the urine which becomes black on standing or when alkalized and this, with the blue-black or dark brown discoloration of ear cartilages, cornea, conjunctiva and skin, particularly the sweat-secreting areas, is the diagnostic giveaway. In addition, wax in the ears may be dark grey-black.

The patient may present with pain and stiffness of the back and restricted rib movement reminiscent of ankylosing spondylitis, but X-rays show normal sacro-iliac joints and calcification of intervertebral discs. Later these discs narrow and disappear, leaving the vertebrae fused together. Knees are affected in many cases but not until ten to twenty years after the backaches started. Hips and shoulders may be affected even later, the joint distribution being bilateral and symmetrical.

The whole arthritic process is so insidious that its nature may not be appreciated if the typical pigmentation of skin and urine are not noticed. This disorder is twice as common in males, joint symptoms starting between twenty and forty in men and between forty and fifty in women.

Treatment Ochronosis is one of the many causes of secondary osteoarthrosis, and the symptomatic treatment is as for that condition.

Familial Mediterranean fever

This is one of the diseases which were previously confined to other parts of the world but are now appearing in our clinics and consulting rooms as a result of increased air travel.

I have seen three cases during the last year, one of whom was aged twenty, of Armenian stock from Iran. There was no relevant family history, which is unusual because the disease is inherited as an autosomal recessive. Since early childhood he had had bouts of abdominal pain and fever lasting two to three days, sometimes with vomiting and/or diarrhoea. Acute painful episodes in hip or knee started when he was fifteen and a half and occurred monthly until he began to take colchicine 0.6 mg twice daily. Since then he has had no more pains apart from one severe attack of pain in the hip which occurred when he had stopped taking colchicine. I found no abnormal signs and so long as he takes his colchicine all should be well.

The usual history in these cases is of attacks of fever with pains in the abdomen, chest and a single joint, usually a knee but sometimes an ankle, hip, elbow or shoulder. Pain may be mild or severe, usually lasting for a few days but sometimes for weeks or months, usually with complete resolution between attacks. The onset is usually in childhood. Both sexes are affected. The joint condition is usually an arthralgia rather than an arthritis, but small effusions are common.

Some 30 per cent of patients develop amyloidosis which leads to renal failure in five to ten years. About 30 per cent develop sacro-iliac radiological changes and half of these later show clinical features of ankylosing spondylitis.

Treatment is with colchicine 0.5 mg two or three times daily, regularly and continuously. This will prevent acute attacks in most cases and possibly ward off amyloidosis in some. Corticosteroids are unhelpful.

Sickle cell disease

This is an inherited condition which may be seen in visitors or immigrants. Haemoglobin A is replaced by haemoglobin S. Heterozygotes who have two different allelomorphic genes in the same locus on each pair of chromosomes are not anaemic or arthritic. Homozygotes with identical genes become severely anaemic and have thrombotic crises which cause bone infarcts with secondary arthritis.

This condition occurs in Blacks, usually in Africa but sometimes elsewhere. The onset is in childhood, with transient swelling, tenderness and pain occurring most often in the hands and feet from periostitis of metacarpals, metatarsals and proximal phalanges (sickle cell dactylitis). Other joints may be affected. X-rays show periosteal elevation and subperiosteal new bone, with a patchy moth-eaten appearance of the bones.

The joint manifestations are usually symmetrical and polyarticular and may be migratory resembling rheumatic fever. Arthralgia is more common than arthritis but the joints may be swollen, red, warm and tender, sometimes with effusions. Bone and back pains may be severe and febrile crises may be precipitated by infection. Attacks may subside within a few days but may then recur. Abdominal pain may simulate an acute surgical emergency. Chronic anaemia with intermittent jaundice is common and leg ulcers or cholelithiasis occur in around one-third of cases. Osteomyelitis is common, often in multiple sites and often due to salmonella. Diagnosis is by demonstration of sickling and by haemoglobin diaphoresis.

Treatment No specific treatment is available. Antibiotics may be needed to treat intercurrent infections, but transfusion of blood may increase viscosity and precipitate further vascular occlusion. Folic acid 1 mg daily is advisable. Analgesics may be given as necessary. Intravenous bicarbonate infusions are sometimes helpful. Hydration must be maintained by intravenous fluids and oxygen must be given as required. No agent has been shown to abort or shorten a painful crisis where symptoms are due to ischaemia and infarction.

Behçet's disease

This disease of unknown origin is characterized by oral and genital ulceration with iritis. Arthritis occurs in 60 per cent of cases. The disease is twice as common in males and starts between the ages of twenty and forty.

Pain and swelling of several joints occurs most often in knees and ankles, less often in elbows, wrists, hands and feet. Effusions are not uncommon. The arthritis is either chronic or intermittent. Alimentary symptoms (diarrhoea, abdominal pain, nausea and anorexia) occur in 50 per cent; skin ulcers, sepsis or erythema nodosum in 65 per cent; and venous thrombosis in 25 per cent. The most serious and sometimes fatal symptoms are the neurological manifestations (headaches, confusion, fits, paralyses or coma) which occur in 10 per cent.

The course is very variable and the prognosis for eventual recovery is usually good, though occasional fatalities may be associated with vascular, gastro-intestinal or neurological complications.

Treatment is symptomatic. Steroids may be helpful.

Needle punctures should be avoided if possible as they may be followed by inflammatory skin lesions.

PRACTICAL POINT

● The main practical point is that while the diagnosis of these unusual arthropathies requires considerable experience and knowledge, once diagnosed there is no specific curative treatment for any of them.

17
Fibrositis: does it exist?

According to Copeman[1] the term 'fibrositis' was coined by Sir William Gowers to include all forms of nonarticular rheumatism, in the belief that they were inflammatory. This belief seemed to be confirmed in 1920 by Stockman in Glasgow.[2] He said that inflammation occurred in fibrous tissue under the skin, particularly around the shoulder girdle and in the lower part of the back. After examining biopsy material he thought he had found histological evidence of such a process and that it was probably infective in origin, although he grew no micro-organisms from the lesions.

Medical mythology

Stockman's findings have not been confirmed by others. No pathological process has been found in further biopsy material and EMGs, serology and ESRs have been normal. Copeman and Ackerman[3] found that the lumps, which are sometimes palpated and may be tender, but are often symptomless, were fatty nodules which had herniated through the fibrous capsules that invested them. Recently Smythe[4] described the 'fibrositis syndrome' as a 'pain magnification state'. The essential clinical features were the presence of large numbers of tender areas in muscle, bone, fibrous tissue and subcutaneous fat, with widespread but poorly localized pains and stiffness, exhaustion and disturbances of sleep. He does not consider the pain magnification to be psychological in origin but describes it as a quantitative change in physiologically normal pain mechanisms.

It is true that aches are common in those areas and that lumps can often be palpated but there is no evidence that any inflammatory change exists in muscles or connective tissue. Physiotherapists have often claimed to have broken up and destroyed nodules with relief of pain, but such claims are somewhat impressionistic even if it is possible that fibrofatty nodules may be fragmented by deep palpation with relief of symptoms.

Diffuse aches, mainly in the back and shoulder girdles, commonly occur after excessive and unusual muscular exertion but rarely also in polymyalgia rheumatica (see Chapter

13), in disseminated connective tissue disorders such as polymyositis, polyarteritis nodosa and systemic lupus erythematosus, and with low-grade infections such as subacute bacterial endocarditis and abortus, melitensis, typhoid and paratyphoid fevers. The late Philip Hench also postulated a fibrositic phase in rheumatoid arthritis, believing that the fibrositic aches preceded or accompanied early rheumatoid changes.

In other cases the pains are probably referred from injury or strain in the spine, usually the dorsal spine, and are merely the symptoms of everyday life, symptoms which may seem more formidable when the pain threshold is lowered by poor health, lack of sleep or adverse emotional or environmental circumstances. The patient is seldom unduly incapacitated or worried, and the diagnosis of 'fibrositis' often brings reassurance because it is generally considered to be a 'nuisance' condition, not at all serious and sure to get better. He would be much more worried if he thought he had lumbago or a slipped disc.

The term is a most useful one to cover lack of medical knowledge of many common aches and pains that are self-limiting and self-resolving. Whatever the true nature of these, the patients come for help and relief, and the physician has to make some attempts at a pathological explanation and a diagnostic label, hence 'fibrositis'.

COMMONSENSE APPROACH

Since this is a benign syndrome with many possible causes and no known pathological basis it does not deserve the status of a 'medical' diagnosis. Better to regard it as a lay term which doctors find useful when they want a name for a collection of aches that will probably go away. Its diminished standing as a proper disease is exemplified in Copeman's *Textbook of the Rheumatic Diseases*. The first edition (1948) had forty-three references to fibrositis. The fifth edition (1978)[5] has one reference.

PRACTICAL POINTS

- It is the essence of general practice that many common aches and pains cannot be accurately diagnosed or pathologically explained, particularly those in the neck, shoulder and back regions.
- As a pseudodiagnosis 'fibrositis' serves:
  1. To offer the patient a real, respectable disease to explain his/her symptoms.
  2. As a useful entry on a medical certificate.
  3. As a good smokescreen to cover medical ignorance.
- It must be understood by the medical profession, however, that it has no basis as a medical fact, and it must be used honestly for what it is, 'medical fiction'.

18
Rheumatic nondisease

Symptoms apparently relating to muscle, bone and joint may be due to organic disease, mental disorder or a combination of both. They can also be due to neither.

PSYCHE

Emotions are not abnormal reactions. Someone who is in love, in despair or bereaved may temporarily be deranged but cannot be said to be diseased. The malingerer produces symptoms for personal reasons, often financial, but many people without any serious disorder find that it pays to have symptoms, and what might be called 'rheumatic nondisease' can be used to gain sympathy from doctors, family and friends; priority in queues; extra attention on bus, train or aeroplane; or even to provide material for conversation.

ACCIDENT NEUROSES

The symptoms may begin with an accident, often at work or on the road, and since the accident was emotionally as well as physically disturbing it becomes an important event in the life of the sufferer, a point in time to which many events are related. With uncertainty about a possible case in the courts or before an industrial or appeal tribunal, the symptoms tend to persist. When uncertainty has been banished by a final decision either for or against the claimant, there is often, but by no means invariably, an improvement or even a complete cure, but symptoms have a way of persisting when a disability pension or some other financial reward depends on their persistence.

REWARDS OF THE SICK ROLE

Frank malingering is rare in comparison with a symptomatic hangover or hang-up in a person who has little or no organic or psychological disorder but still feels aggrieved and hard done by. A similar but domestic syndrome can be started at home by an upsetting or demoralizing event. After an injury or during an illness someone finds so much sympathy, care and affection bestowed on him by the rest of the family that symptoms persist in spite of complete recovery from the original disorder. An incident as trivial as a vasovagal attack may completely change the attitude of the whole family to the fainter and lead to endless care and attention being lavished on him.

NONHEALTH OR NONDISEASE

Although there may be a very narrow dividing line between nondisease and a psychiatric disorder such as depression or an anxiety state, Prof Szasz[1] is probably correct when he says that in these modern times everything has to be explained in terms of disease. We are not allowed to explain disorders in terms of normal though perhaps exaggerated emotional responses or attitudes of mind.

Disorders of the locomotor system are copious in this no-man's land, this limbo between disease and full health. The usual aches and pains that are the everyday lot of all of us can be magnified by unhappiness or an upsetting event into symptoms that usually relate to the cervical or lumbar spine but sometimes to other areas in the locomotor system.

It is all too easy for doctors to create nondisease. A raised uric acid, for instance, is too frequently taken to signify gout when the trouble is due to other, simpler conditions such as bad shoes or osteoarthrosis of the big toe. Once gout has been announced to be present and become, as it were, official, the sufferer rises in family and social prestige, especially if he has been put on to allopurinol or some other drug for a period pronounced to be indefinite. From now on the patient and perhaps his doctor may ascribe many unrelated symptoms to his main but nonexistent disease.

A similar state of affairs may follow a misdiagnosis of osteoarthrosis or even of rheumatoid arthritis. Lives may be completely changed, homes sold in favour of new ones in warmer climes, retirements taken prematurely, engagements broken and contracts terminated. Many people are glad enough to have a medical label which can be used to diplomatic advantage in a variety of circumstances and the titles 'rheumatism' and 'arthritis' can become escape hatches from difficult situations even when no real disability exists. The fact that X-ray changes are certain to be found in the cervical or lumbar spine of anyone over sixty makes a diagnosis of osteoarthritis especially easy to earn.

THE DANGERS OF MISINTERPRETING INVESTIGATIONS

Special investigations carry their own danger in that they may be misinterpreted in relation to a particular patient. When a new laboratory test is developed there is usually a period of months or years before its practical application to clinical medicine is quite clearly cut.

The discovery that the tissue antigen HLAB27 is present in some 95 per cent of people with ankylosing spondylitis in Great Britain was a very useful step towards an understanding of this disease, but it is not a diagnostic investigation. Eight per cent of the population have this antigen and many of them will have backache, but it is still unlikely that they will develop ankylosing spondylitis, which is much less common than other causes of pain in the back.

THE IMPORTANCE OF HISTORY-TAKING

The diagnosis of nondisease depends on careful history-taking and physical examination more than on investigations which often mislead. The history of one of the usual rheumatic disorders takes familiar shape as it is related and forms a pattern which usually suggests a diagnosis. In nondisease, however, the history is bizarre and unusual apart from a few cases so classical that they seem to have come straight out of a book.

A few deliberately misleading questions may help to detect nondisease, the patient readily admitting to nonsensical symptoms as part of his syndrome. Difficulties may arise with patients who speak little or no English because interpreters often mislead unintentionally or even intentionally by rephrasing questions and answers in a way that they think may be helpful.

In the old days such exaggeration of symptoms was typical of hysteria, but hysteria is now a rare disorder in developed countries and hysterical features are absent in these patients who seldom exhibit paralysis or anaesthesia.

HOW TO DETECT NONDISEASE DURING EXAMINATION

Examination usually confirms the impression given by the history. Movements are often restricted to a degree far in excess of that found in any disorder known to medicine. When the patient is asked to move the painful joint both flexors and extensors go into action and when passive movement is attempted there is resistance in all muscle groups, but when the patient's attention is diverted to other parts of his body a greater range of passive movement becomes possible. If he is encouraged to make explanatory gestures active movements are greater than those that seemed possible during examination.

The nondiseased patient's history and behaviour on examination are a conscious or half-conscious demonstration of the severity, the awfulness of his condition and the badness of his 'bad' joint. They are intended to impress. Words like 'agony' and 'terrible' flow from his lips and pain and dysfunction are to be found in muscles and tissues quite unrelated to the part of which he complains.

THE SEX EVASION SYNDROME

Two female patients of mine had severe pain in the hip during sexual intercourse and this prevented normal marital relations with their husbands. Both were in their thirties. In each case the marriage appeared to be happy though childless.

In neither case were there any positive investigations or abnormal X-ray findings, nor did any develop during a three-year follow up. The only positive physical sign was moderate discomfort during a full range of movement of the hip. Although it is possible that an early capsulitis was present this did not affect hip function in any other way: walking, standing and ascending and descending steps were carried out normally and painlessly. I was left with the impression that these were cases of an evasion syndrome, a domestic variant of nondisease.

PRACTICAL POINTS

● Psyche can produce a whole range of rheumatic symptoms.
● Accident neurosis is not uncommon when compensation is under negotiation.
● Doctors often create nondisease by misinterpreting signs and results of investigations.

19
Pain

BACKGROUND

Pain varies greatly with the personality of the sufferer. Pain also varies greatly in its significance to that sufferer. Pain is always unpleasant but it may also be ominous, bringing anxiety and fear. For many people pain may be a call for action, with treatment expected and immediate relief demanded whenever any pain is felt in any part of the body, but there are other people who have been brought up to think of pain as part of living, something that has to be accepted and borne.

Sociocultural factors

There are different racial, tribal and familial attitudes to pain. These are exemplified by a Nigerian friend's observation of people in three different areas of his own country. In one area it is bad form to talk about pain or even to mention it and such operations as the lancing of an abscess or the setting of a fracture must be endured without complaint. In another area it is completely acceptable to talk about pain, which is a popular topic of conversation. These people expect a local anaesthetic. In a third area patients will tolerate pain and submit to operations without anaesthetic provided the doctor is pleasant and apologizes in advance.

Added anxiety and depression

Generally speaking any pain that lasts for days or weeks is often accompanied by anxiety, while one that lasts much longer becomes tinged with depression and this depression may come to be a large part of the painful syndrome.

In the early stages of a disease such as rheumatoid arthritis treatment of anxiety may be helpful, but once the patient has passed into the next depressive phase reassurance and other anti-anxiety measures may be worse than useless because they not only fail to relieve the patient but may also make him lose confidence in his doctor.

The constitutionally depressed patient, who readily becomes depressed or down-hearted, tends to suffer pain more severely than someone with a more buoyant personality, but a long-lasting pain is likely to bring depression to everyone. Depression alone is capable of causing pain or mental anguish that cannot always be readily distinguished from other types of pain. Such depressive pains are more likely to occur in the back, head and neck than in the extremities. Depression sometimes leads to the resurrection of pains in places where organic disease once put them.

Wider significance

Pain therefore acquires a symbolic aspect and a meaning quite apart from the arthritic disorder that is causing it. It may be an appeal for sympathy on the patient's behalf, it may betoken a desire for more attention, it may be meant to stimulate a feeling of guilt in those around, but it may, in some cases, act to purge the patient's own sense of guilt. It has even been said that pain can offer an escape from depression which would cause more suffering than the pain itself. An arthritic pain that is accompanied by depression may also be accompanied by lethargy, tension, fatiguability and sleep disturbance, all of which are often attributed to the painful joint condition, when in reality they are due to depression.

Hysteria

Hysteria is now a rarity. Hysterics may manipulate others emotionally and the hysterical patient often overreacts to produce dramatic symptoms.

Hypochondria

In hypochondriasis the patient is fascinated and absorbed by his painful experiences. In one study of hypochondriasis 70 per cent had pain and of these, 55 per cent had headaches, 20 per cent had chest pains and 16 per cent had abdominal pains. Pain in joints is less common. Since hypochondriacs are enthralled by illness they welcome investigations and like to have them repeated.

A doctor who fails to give firm reassurance and explain fully the result of investigations may add to his patient's self-absorbed anxiety. It has been suggested that a hypochondriacal attitude to health is a learned response that developed in childhood, often in a family in which the child could only obtain a favourable response from his parents by being ill.

PAIN IN RHEUMATOID ARTHRITIS

This is a compound of many unpleasant feelings:

- Discomfort from the inflamed and altered joint tissues.
- General malaise, with fever and anaemia.
- Depression and anxiety, with anger at being unable to perform simple functions without help.
- Ill effects of drugs.
- Symptoms due to nonarticular features of rheumatoid disease, including arteritis, neuropathies, crush fractures of vertebrae, pleurisy and pericarditis.

Pain thresholds vary, and the point at which a stimulus becomes a pain differs between one person and another. A patient's pain threshold may be roughly estimated as average, high or low by pressing the forehead with an algiometer. A low-threshold person will have more pain and take more analgesics while someone with a high threshold will be less discommoded by disease of apparently similar severity. While a particular person's threshold remains fairly steady the severity of his arthritic symptoms may be made to fluctuate by depression, anxiety or other pains.

ANTIDEPRESSANTS

The addition of an antidepressant drug will produce symptomatic improvement in many patients with rheumatoid arthritis even when there is no demonstrable change in the joints. There are many antidepressants, some of which act quickly, while others, such as imipramine, do not begin to be effective until two to three weeks have passed. Some, such as amitriptyline, have an immediate sedative effect even though the antidepressive effect is delayed.

Antidepressants

Generic name	Dosage
amitriptyline	50–100 mg nocte or 75 mg daily in divided dosage.
butriptyline	25–50 mg × 3 daily.
clomipramine	10–50 mg nocte or in divided dosage by day.
desipramine	25–50 mg × 3 daily.
dothiepin	75–150 mg nocte or in divided dose in the day.
doxepin	10–100 mg nocte or 10–100 mg × 3 daily.
flupenthioxol	0.5–1 mg × 2–3 daily.
imipramine	25–50 mg × 3 daily.
iprindole	15–30 mg × 3 daily.
iproniazid*	25–150 mg daily as single dose.
isocarboxazid*	10–30 mg daily.
l-tryptophan	1,000 mg × 3 daily.
maprotiline	25–75 mg nocte or in divided dosage in day. Maximum 150 mg daily.
mianserin	30–40 mg nocte or in divided dosage by day.
nomifensine	75–200 mg daily in divided dosage.
nortriptyline	10–25 mg × 3–4 daily.
protriptyline	15–60 mg daily in divided dosage up to 90 mg or more.
tofenacin	80–240 mg in divided dosage.
trazodone	100–150 mg nocte or in divided dosage in the day. Maximum 600 mg daily.
trimipramine	50–75 mg 2 hours before retiring.
viloxazine	50–100 mg × 3 daily.
phenelzine*	15 mg × 1–3 daily.
tranylcypromine*	10 mg × 1–3 daily.

*These are monoamine oxidase inhibitors (MAOIs) and are subject to the usual dietetic restrictions and other precautions.

The choice of an antidepressant must depend on the needs of the particular patient. While amitriptyline is good when sedation is needed, imipramine is adequate if sedation seems unnecessary. The Table opposite lists useful antidepressants.

All drugs in the Table should be used with caution in cardiovascular and liver disorders, epilepsy, diabetes and patients with known suicidal tendencies. All, except mianserin, should be used with extreme caution in conditions where an anticholinergic agent would be undesirable (eg, glaucoma, urinary retention, pyloric stenosis or prostatic hypertrophy). Interactions with other drugs may occur, particularly with alcohol, MAOIs, anticholinergic agents and local anaesthetics containing noradrenaline.

PRACTICAL POINTS

- Persistent pain leads to loss of morale, anxiety and depression.
- Management of depression may produce improvement, even if pain persists.
- Holistic management of the patient is essential.

20

Rashes in rheumatology

BACKGROUND

Skin and joints have a close relationship. Many rheumatological conditions have skin rashes as part of their clinical syndrome, and many primary skin disorders also involve joints and connective tissues. In addition, iatrogenic rashes may occur from side-effects of the drugs used to treat rheumatic conditions.

When associated with rheumatological disorders, rashes present intriguing diagnostic challenges to the clinician.

DIAGNOSTIC RASHES

These are found in the following conditions.

Psoriatic arthropathy

Even small patches of psoriasis may point to the true diagnosis of an arthropathy that may affect many joints or only a few. The typical scaly patches, which look silvery when scratched, may be diffuse all over the body, including all the limbs, or confined to one or two small patches of skin. If there are only a few skin patches they are most likely to be found on the scalp at the hair margin, over the upper tibia just below the patella, or on the extensor surface of the forearm, just below the elbow.

The patient has usually been aware of his psoriasis for several years before the development of arthritis, but it occasionally happens that he has not noticed the skin condition or has thought it too trivial to mention. The discovery of a few small spots may solve the problem in a case of seronegative arthritis or of back pain with sacro-iliac changes. (See also Chapter 8.)

Reiter's disease

This may produce keratoderma blennorrhagica. The skin lesions, particularly the hard scaly rash on the soles of the feet, are often very similar to those of psoriasis and cannot always be distinguished from it histologically. At an early stage of this rash there may be vesicles which have an erythematous base and develop into sterile pustules. Keratotic plaques and papules occur on the skin of the scalp and elsewhere.

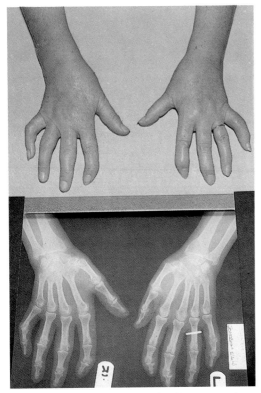

Figure 61 Psoriatic arthropathy showing patchy
involvement of all finger joints. The finger nails are
affected by psoriasis. The left terminal interphalangeal
joint of the index finger is acutely inflamed and
subluxated.

Mouth ulcers are common and there may be vesicular or papular lesions on the penis.
Such lesions may be mistaken for syphilitic chancres. The probable diagnosis should be
indicated by a history of venereal exposure or dysentery with acute arthropathy
principally affecting ankles and knees and coexisting with urethritis and often
conjunctivitis. (See also page 43).

Bacteraemia

Purulent skin lesions may coexist with septic arthritis (pyarthrosis) as in staphylococcal,
meningococcal, gonococcal or streptococcal septicaemia.

Gonococcal   In these cases skin lesions occur as crops of pustular, maculopapular,
haemorrhagic or vesicular lesions. The pyarthrosis may involve one to four joints, the
knee being most commonly affected. Positive bacterial culture from blood, skin or
joint is necessary for diagnosis. The gonococcal complement fixation test is unreliable
because it gives false positives as well as false negatives.

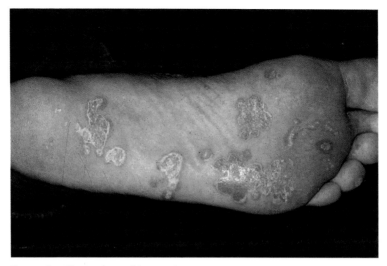

Figure 62   Keratoderma blennorrhagica in Reiter's disease.

Meningococcal infection may be epidemic or sporadic and may occur with or without meningitis. Purpura is common. The arthritis may be septic or it may be reactive, without suppuration.

Systemic lupus erythematosus

There is some type of skin reaction in 75 per cent of cases. It may take a macular, papular, discoid, purpuric or almost any other form. The most characteristic but not the most common is a heliotrope rash – in the shape of a butterfly with its body on the nose and its wings on the cheeks – which occurs in the more acute phases of the disease.

Another diagnostic skin lesion is a circumscribed and slightly indurated purplish-red plaque. Both hyper- and hypopigmentation may occur as may telangiectases, scaling and skin atrophy. Such rashes may be localized or they may be diffuse and may occur anywhere on the trunk, extremities or scalp. Alopecia and photosensitivity may also occur.

Dermatomyositis

The most characteristic rash is a purple-red discoloration and oedema of the eyelids, with erythematous macules, scaling occurring on head, feet and upper trunk, with purple-red papules which develop into atrophic plaques with pigmentary changes and telangiectases. These lesions are particularly likely to be found on the backs of the knuckles.

Juvenile chronic polyarthritis (Still's disease)

There may be a transient erythematous rash. Small erythematous lesions, macules or

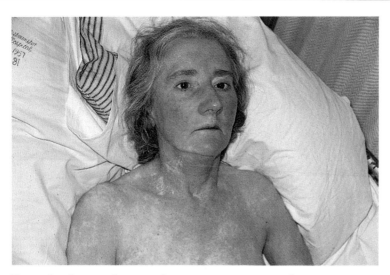

Figure 63   Systemic lupus erythematosus in acute exacerbation.

papules over face, trunk and extremities, may come with active phases of the disease and disappear as the arthritis improves. (See also Chapter 11.)

Rheumatic fever

Erythema marginatum appears as pink rings usually with red margins and spreads rapidly peripherally to reach a diameter of 2–10 mm in half a day.

Erythema circinata is a flat or macular form of skin reaction. These skin lesions are often associated with active carditis.

Erythema nodosum over the front of the shins is associated with sarcoidosis and a number of other conditions (see page 126).

TOXIC RASHES

There is probably no drug in general use that is not capable of causing some sort of rash in some patients. The antirheumatics are no exception. The following are the antirheumatic drugs prescribed in general practice that most often induce skin rashes.

Gold salts

Skin rashes occur in about a third of patients treated with gold salts and are the commonest reason for having to stop treatment.

Rashes may range in severity from mild erythema to unpleasant pruritus and through to lethal exfoliative dermatitis. They may resemble many different skin diseases including psoriasis, lichen planus, pityriasis rosea and, rarely, erythema nodosum.

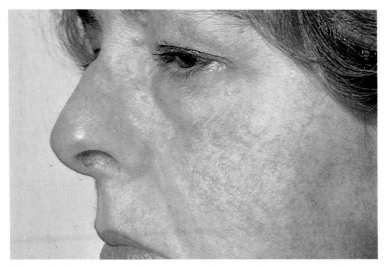

Figure 64 Dermatomyositis, showing rash on the face and nose and periorbital oedema.

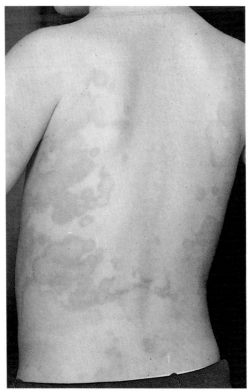

Figure 65 Erythema marginatum in a child with rheumatic fever.

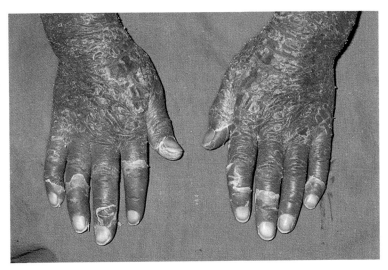

Figure 66 Exfoliative dermatitis in a black African subject.

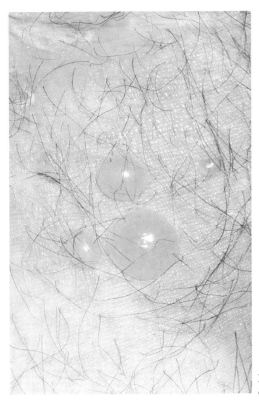

Figure 67 Pemphigoid reaction (see overleaf).

Penicillamine

Reactions to this drug may occur early, within two months of starting treatment, or later, after about a year's continuous therapy. In the former case it may be possible to restart the drug at a lower dosage, but in the latter it is unwise to do so because there have been some very severe reactions on restarting.

Rashes are the commonest toxic effects of this agent and may range from a simple erythematous, macular, papular or urticarial rash to a pemphigoid type of reaction.

Antimalarials

Skin reactions to chloroquine and hydroxychloroquine have seldom proved serious although there may be depigmentation of the hair, mobilliform or maculopapular rashes and, rarely, exfoliation and desquamation.

Allopurinol

This drug is used for the long-term prophylaxis of gout. Skin rashes, sometimes with fever, have been reported in 2.1 per cent of patients given allopurinol alone, but in 22.4 per cent of those given allopurinol and ampicillin. It is obvious that the two drugs should not be given at the same time.

In giving any treatment that may be continued for years, it is always necessary to keep the possibility of drug interactions in mind. Although allopurinol may rarely cause swelling and intense itching of the body and sometimes the face it is usually possible to restart the drug at a reduced dosage after temporary discontinuation.

NSAIDs

The NSAID most commonly responsible for rashes was alclofenac which has now been withdrawn for that reason. Fenclofenac and feprazone have been reported as causing skin rashes in 7–10 per cent of patients; both have been withdrawn in the UK.

A variety of skin reactions, some severe and including the Stevens-Johnson syndrome (see below), have been reported with phenylbutazone and other NSAIDs. Phenylbutazone, the earliest of these drugs, was first marketed in 1952 and the longer a drug has been in use the more likely it is to have been the subject of adverse reports. It (phenylbutazone) has now been withdrawn in Great Britain except for hospital treatment of ankylosing spondylitis.

Of the newer preparations benoxaprofen causes light-sensitivity reactions and produces nail separation (onycholysis) in over 8–12 per cent of patients. It has now been withdrawn. Fenbufen causes skin reactions in 4–5 per cent or more of cases.

No NSAID is quite immune from causing skin rashes but most if not all of these drugs affect the gastro-intestinal tract more often than the skin. (See Chapter 29.)

THE STEVENS-JOHNSON SYNDROME

This was first described in the United States in 1922. It is a diffuse form of severe erythema multiforme with fever, inflammation of the buccal mucosa and purulent conjunctivitis. The syndrome has a mortality rate of 1–10 per cent, according to different reports from different parts of the world.

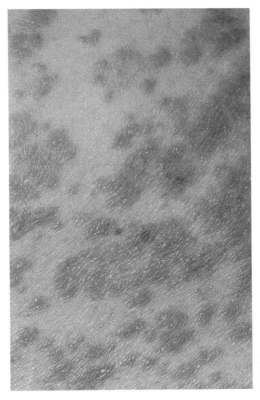

Figure 68 Rash in erythema multiforme (Stevens-Johnson syndrome) due
to drug reaction.

When it is caused by drugs, as it is in 80 per cent of cases, one of the penicillins or
long-acting sulpha drugs is usually at fault, but aspirin or phenylbutazone may be
responsible, and some of the more recently marketed NSAIDs have been blamed in a
few reports.

Gold salts are a rare cause of this syndrome.

Dermatitis artefacta

It should not be forgotten that skin rashes can be produced by the patient for a number
of reasons, either to stay in hospital longer, to gain more sympathy and attention, or
for obscure psychiatric reasons. Blisters may be produced with cigarette ends,
scratches may be aggravated by salt or pepper rubbed into the area; pinching and bruising
can also be produced. A significant feature of dermatitis artefacta is that it occurs
within the reach of the patient's arms. It is therefore rare between the scapulae and
areas which cannot be approached except with long-handled instruments. Gross
oedema of the hands and arm and of the leg can be produced by tightening pyjama
trousers round the thigh or nightdresses around the tops of the arms.

PRACTICAL POINTS

● **Skin disorders associated with joint lesions**
 —Psoriasis – seronegative arthritis or sacro-iliitis.
 —Reiter's disease – polymorphic skin lesions on soles of feet, mouth ulcers, urethritis, conjunctivitis and acute arthritis of knees and ankles.
● **Joint disorders associated with skin lesions**
 —Juvenile chronic polyarthritis – transient erythema.
 —Rheumatic fever – erythematous rashes.
● **Bacteraemia (with pustules and rashes)**
 —Staphylococcal
 —Meningococcal
 —Gonococcal
 —Streptococcal
● **Systemic connective tissue (collagen) disorders with joint and skin problems**
 —Systemic lupus erythematosus
 —Dermatomyositis
● **Toxic drug rashes**
 —Gold salts
 —Penicillamine
 —Antimalarials
 —Allopurinol
 —NSAIDs
 —Immunoregulatory drugs (not usually prescribed in general practice)
● **Dermatitis artefacta should never be forgotten.**

21
Dyspepsia and arthritis

BACKGROUND

Combinations of dyspepsia with some form of arthritis are unpleasant and common. NSAIDs tend to aggravate or initiate dyspepsia, probably if only partly because they suppress the protective action of prostaglandins on the gastric mucosa (see also Chapter 29). It is also possible that rheumatoid patients are more prone to dyspepsia than other people, but it is difficult to be sure of this because most of them have already had a good deal of treatment before they are investigated.

FREQUENCY

Barium studies have revealed a somewhat greater prevalence of gastric ulcers in patients on NSAIDs as compared with others. Use of modern flexible endoscopes has gone further than the mere confirmation of this finding. It has shown that irritative gastric changes and duodenal and other intestinal lesions are more frequent and more severe than had been thought.

Using an oblique-viewing gastroduodenoscope (Olympus GIF-K), Caruso and Bianchi Porro found a number of superficial erosions or ulcers in 164 rheumatoid and 85 osteoarthrotic patients who had been taking antirheumatic drugs continuously for between three and six months.[1]

They found erosions or ulcers in:

- —50 per cent (13 of 26) on aspirin
- —40 per cent (2 of 5) on indoprofen
- —30 per cent (6 of 20) on indomethacin
- —27 per cent (3 of 11) on naproxen
- —20 per cent (2 of 10) on diclofenac
- —18 per cent (3 of 17) on ibuprofen
- —15 per cent (2 of 13) on oxyphenbutazone
- —14 per cent (3 of 21) on corticosteroids
- —11 per cent (2 of 19) on sulindac
- —10 per cent (2 of 20) on diflunisal
- —0 per cent on injections of corticotrophin

Gastric lesions were found in 23 per cent of patients (41 of 177) treated with a single drug, but in 51 per cent (37 of 72) of those who were receiving two or more.

Objective findings did not mirror symptoms and the patients' complaints gave little indication of what was found at gastroscopy. In all cases endoscopy had been normal before treatment was begun. There were no histological studies.

Lanza studied the effects of various NSAIDs on forty healthy volunteers.[2] After seven days no irritative lesions were seen in those taking an inert placebo. The most marked changes were seen in those taking aspirin (3.6 g daily) and symptoms were usually present in those who showed endoscopic abnormalities. Naproxen (750 mg daily) and indomethacin (100 or 150 mg) were associated with similar findings. Ibuprofen (1.6 g) and naproxen (500 mg) produced significantly fewer changes.

ASPIRIN EFFECTS

Aspirin, like many NSAIDs, causes gastro-intestinal symptoms, but the reported incidence varies between 2 per cent and nearly 40 per cent, depending on how the survey was done and on whether the patients knew they were having aspirin. In several controlled trials aspirin and buffered aspirin have been found equally likely to cause symptoms.

In drug trials where a new NSAID has been compared with aspirin, gastro-intestinal symptoms, quite apart from endoscopic findings, are almost always more marked and more common in the aspirin-treated patients.

Local or topical?

An important question is whether this gastric irritation is a local effect of the drug on the mucosa, a blood-borne toxic effect of the drug after it has been absorbed, or a mixture of both.

Douthwaite and Lintott (1938)[3] showed that aspirin has a strong local effect. Thirteen of sixteen subjects showed gastro-intestinal irritation, and in some cases fragments of tablets were embedded in swollen and inflamed gastric mucosa. Their findings have been confirmed by many other workers.

There are many forms of aspirin but most endoscopic studies have been done with regular pharmacopoeial preparations. A two-week, single-blind, crossover trial by Hoftiezer et al,[4] using nine healthy volunteers, showed that all subjects taking 2.4 g of ordinary aspirin daily developed multiple gastric erosions but that only two subjects taking enteric-coated capsules developed one erosion each. Five subjects developed duodenal erosions on regular aspirin but none developed them when taking the coated preparation. A period of two treatment-free weeks separated each two periods of treatment. Mean fasting levels of serum salicylate were similar with both preparations. This is not always the case when regular and enteric-coated aspirin preparations are compared. These authors concluded that the topical effects of aspirin are more important than the systemic effects as a cause of mucosal damage in healthy subjects.

Other workers have shown that intravenous aspirin dosage sufficient to produce the same serum salicylate levels as oral dosage caused only a negligible increase of faecal blood loss as compared with that of other healthy subjects taking a placebo.[5,6] This again suggests that a local action is involved.

Blood loss

Faecal blood loss is greater with aspirin than with other NSAIDs, but it is usually so slight that the ordinary occult blood tests are negative. Blood loss can only be revealed by special investigations that involve the use of radioactive isotopes. Average blood loss in normal untreated subjects is about 0.5 ml a day but it is around 2.5 ml in 70 per cent of people on aspirin with an occasional patient losing as much as 16 ml. Alcohol increases the tendency to microbleeding.[7,8] However, it is rarely sufficient to influence treatment or to cause anaemia, even if it contributes to it in some cases.

According to Plotz,[9] salicylate compounds can be divided into two groups:

1. **About equivalent in ability to cause blood loss** In this group are aspirin, soluble aspirin, calcium aspirin, aspirin in solution or suspension, aspirin given with milk, some enteric-coated aspirins and some over-the-counter buffered aspirins.[10–12]

2. **Causing little or no blood loss** These include sodium salicylate, choline salicylate, effervescent aspirin, aspirin given with enough sodium bicarbonate and aspirin given with enough of a nonabsorbable, nonsodium buffer.

When it comes to assessing how often more serious and obvious bleeding occurs I agree with Plotz when he says that some cases of major gastro-intestinal bleeding or ulceration are related to recent ingestion of aspirin and with Spiro[13] when he says that aspirin is dangerous to the peptic ulcer patient even though it probably only causes superficial erosions.

Although chronic duodenal ulceration may be aggravated by aspirin there is little evidence that it is initiated by aspirin alone. As regards gastric ulceration, Levy[14] found that habitual administration of aspirin did contribute to the causation of benign ulcer and to episodes of bleeding. He estimated that the drug added a total of 25 cases per 100,000 users per annum.

There seems to be no doubt that aspirin is the most irritant of the NSAIDs in general use but that the superficial erosions and haemorrhages are often, perhaps usually, unaccompanied by symptoms and are an acceptable price to pay for relief of pain, swelling and stiffness.

PATIENT COMPLIANCE

Few arthritic patients select aspirin as their first choice of a drug for long-term treatment. A large majority prefer a drug which can be taken less frequently and which causes less dyspepsia, tinnitus and deafness. Compliance is better when fewer daily doses are needed and a number of NSAIDs which are now available only need to be taken once or twice a day.

Forty-five patients with osteoarthrosis were the subject of a study reported at the Ninth European Congress on Rheumatism (Wiesbaden, 1979).[15] Over a two-week period they took Voltarol (enteric-coated diclofenac), 25 mg in the morning, 25 mg at noon and 50 mg at bedtime, and for a further two weeks they took one 100 mg slow-release pill of the same agent, once a day only. In the first period 87 doses (2,075 mg) were missed and in the second period only 12 (1,200 mg). Compliance was 45 per cent better with the once-daily slow-release formulation. While 25 patients preferred the single dose, only 2 preferred the thrice-daily regime. It is often said that the mere taking of medicine has a therapeutic effect and this may be true in some circumstances such as those of a short-term illness which will soon get better in any event or when anxiety is an important feature. It does not seem to be true in chronic painful conditions such as osteo- or rheumatoid arthritis. Where treatment is mainly symptomatic, the patient who feels he can skip a dose may not need it.

WHAT TO DO?

The possibility of causing gastro-intestinal symptoms is present with all the NSAIDs. Though some appear to cause more irritation than others, none are entirely free from this hazard. Antacids may ease symptoms but this may mask underlying disease. Cimetidine is of great assistance. It can induce healing and reduce symptoms even when NSAIDs have to be continued because the patient's arthritis does not allow his antirheumatic drug to be withdrawn. There is evidence that it has a protective effect on aspirin-related gastric damage[16] and reduces gastro-intestinal bleeding from this cause.[17] Nevertheless in the presence of acute dyspeptic symptoms or of gastro-intestinal irritation or bleeding, it is usually wise, if humanly possible, to discontinue or reduce the NSAID dosage in the hope of preventing a more serious complication such as perforation or further haemorrhage.

The dyspeptic arthritic is one of the most difficult patients to treat and although cimetidine, ranitidine, and other agents have made it easier to cope with, major surgery such as pyloroplasty and/or vagotomy is often required before adequate drug treatment can be resumed. Just to make life more difficult, there are recent reports that cimetidine itself may cause arthralgia and, rarely, arthritic changes.

PRACTICAL POINTS

- All antirheumatic drugs can cause dyspepsia.
- NSAIDs cause increased incidence of gastric and, less often, duodenal ulcers.
- Aspirin is the most irritant NSAID on stomach, with most faecal blood loss.
- NSAIDs have to be individually tailored to suit the patient.
- Dyspeptic side-effects can be minimized by antacids and perhaps by the receptor antagonists.

22

Instability and falls

BACKGROUND

The elderly population increases every year, with more and more widows and widowers living alone. Instability of the legs often spells doom for these old people, especially when a fall leads to fracture of the neck of the femur, an accident that is always potentially serious and often fatal.

COMMON CAUSES

While common causes of falls include simple faints, drop attacks due to atherosclerotic changes in the carotids, heart block, strokes and ischaemic cardiac episodes, a large number are due to weakness and defects in muscles, bones and joints. The quadriceps muscles may be so feeble that they give way. This is a common cause of drop attacks in the aged and one that is quite unrelated to cardiovascular causes.

RHEUMATIC CAUSES

Pain, swelling and instability of the knees are common in rheumatoid and osteoarthritis and make rapid changes of position or direction impossible. A fixed hip, whatever its cause, leads to abnormal gait and posture, often with shortening of a leg. The rigid neck of ankylosing spondylitis may crack across like a long bone and 60 per cent of such fractures lead to death from injury to the cervical cord.

Enforced inactivity often leads to obesity with further reduction of mobility and stability. Poor sight increases the risk of falls. Impairment of vision may be part of the arthritic syndrome, as in the iritis of ankylosing spondylitis or Reiter's disease and the scleritis or scleromalacia perforans of rheumatoid arthritis.

WHAT TO DO?

What then can be done to deal with this common problem of the patient who is unsteady on the legs because of joint disease?

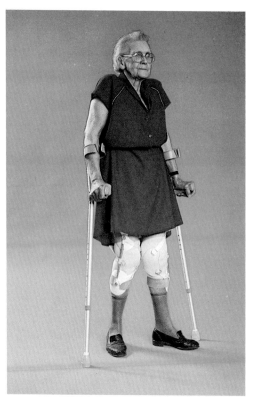

Figure 69a. Elbow crutches help increase mobility when knee supports are needed.

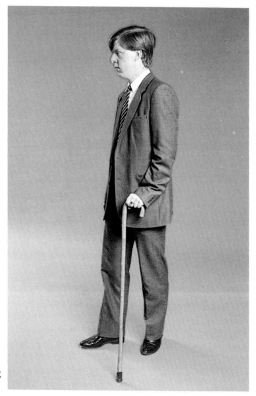

Figure 69b. Correct use of non-skid walking stick.

Figure 69c. Elbow crutches lend stability to patients with built-up footwear.

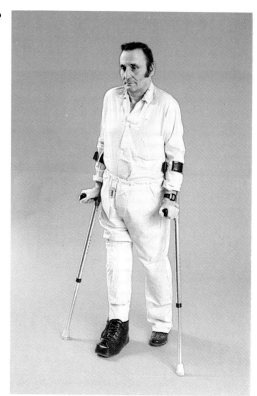

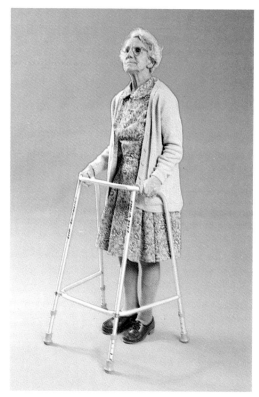

Figure 69d. Walking frames provide support for particularly unstable patients.

1. **Instruct the patient in the art of walking**, moving and exercising in the safest and most effective manner consistent with the disability. Teach the correct use of walking aids, whether sticks, crutches, frames or tripods.

2. **Give advice about safety in the home**   Recommend that rails and extra banisters are fitted. A rail whose cross-section is round and of fairly small diameter is more effective in stimulating the grasp reflex than one whose section is square, rectangular or large. Avoid polished floors and mats that may slip, trip or catch in shoes. Be sure that there is enough light everywhere. Vision is important to the maintenance of an erect posture and the bedroom should never be pitch dark. There should be a light-switch within easy reach of the bed. Many fatal accidents occur when an old person gets up at night to pass water. Try to reduce the need for bending, reaching and climbing.

   Almost every home contains a hundred death traps, even for the healthy. Many can be eliminated after a detailed inspection by an occupational therapist accompanied by the local authority's housing officer or a private builder.

3. **Check footwear**   A chiropodist can help with advice. Shoes should be comfortable and easy to don and doff but they need not be floppy.

4. **Support can be given** with light polythene splints for unstable knees and callipers for foot drop or flail ankles.

5. **Weight of the obese should be reduced**   This is usually much more easily said than done.

6. **Drugs**   Avoid the overuse of sedative drugs by day or night, especially if alcohol has been taken. Long-acting hypnotics such as nitrazepam are less suitable for the elderly than those with a shorter effect such as chlor-methiazole, chloral hydrate or dichlorphenazone. Barbiturates are particularly liable to cause confusion and falls in the night in elderly people and should be avoided.

7. **Emergency help should be easy to call**   A bell or whistle is satisfactory if it can be heard by people who live in the same house or are only separated from it by a thin party wall, but when the patient lives alone the telephone or an alarm bell is of limited use: neither is any good when it is in the sitting room and the patient is lying helpless on the floor of the w.c.

   Some companies provide an emergency-call broadcasting device that can be worn. By pressing a button the wearer is put into contact with a twenty-four-hour monitoring service. This service is expensive, however, and is not available from State-run health services.

Other considerations

The main danger of a fall is a fracture, particularly of the neck of the femur but also of the vertebrae or limbs.

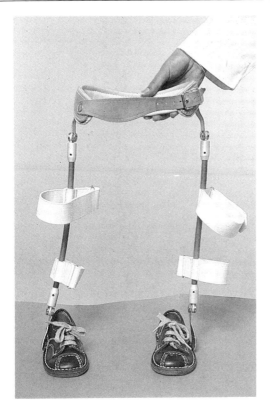

Figure 70 Shoes with fitted callipers, which can be used for foot drop or flail ankles.

Rheumatoid and elderly patients and anyone else who is unable to take exercise are likely to develop osteoporosis and the danger is increased by corticosteroids (see Chapter 30). A multiplicity of hazards combine in the elderly female rheumatoid who is taking corticosteroids and has unstable knees as well as steroid-induced cataracts.

In osteoarthrosis, happily, the necks of the femora have periosteal thickening with strong new bone which makes them unlikely to fracture.

One of my elderly patients, for instance, is eighty-nine years old and lives in an apartment block. Her skeleton is 'overstable' in the sense that she has severe osteoarthrosis with very limited movement in both her hips and the whole of her spine. She is rather deaf but she can call a friend from the ground floor by telephone. She has domestic help every morning, and several friends and a few relations who drop in quite often. Her bathroom, bedroom and other rooms have been modified to suit her needs and she has a high but comfortable armchair. She copes pretty well, for all her disabilities, and like most old people she prefers to live like this with her own things around her rather than go into a home or a geriatric unit.

PRACTICAL POINTS

- Many causes of falls in the elderly, including CVS and CNS causes.
- Rheumatic causes such as instability of knees, arthrosis of hips, and weak thigh muscles probably are more common causes.
- Prevention and management include commonsense advice such as instructions on safety measures, fitting rails at home, avoiding slippery surfaces, and avoidance of sedative drugs.

PART 4: DISEASES WITH RHEUMATIC ASSOCIATIONS

23

Anaemia and other blood disorders

BACKGROUND

Anaemia is commonly associated with rheumatic disorders, and other blood disorders may also be part of the clinical syndromes. Anaemia and other blood disorders that occur in rheumatic disorders may be classified as:

- Those that are part of the actual disease process, as in rheumatoid arthritis.
- Those that may result from side-effects of the drugs being used in treatment.
- Those that may be attributable to diet deficiencies because of the illness or some other reason such as malabsorption.
- Those that may result from blood loss or haemolytic episodes.
- Those that may result from more than one cause.

The practical approach always must be to consider the blood disorder as secondary to some other factor and not to imagine that it is the blood disorder that has to be treated per se.

OSTEOARTHROSIS

Anaemia is no part of the disease process and if it exists it is due to some concurrent malady or to the drugs given. Most of the patients are middle-aged or elderly and more likely than their juniors to suffer from concurrent diseases and to have a poor tolerance for drugs.

RHEUMATOID ARTHRITIS

Anaemia is part of the disease and in the absence of other causal factors the serum iron level is a good measure of its activity. Anaemia is the most common extra-articular manifestation of rheumatoid arthritis and with older patients who suffer a late onset it is well nigh inevitable.

Types of anaemia

The anaemia of rheumatoid arthritis is usually normocytic and normochromic but may be hypochromic and normocytic, unlike iron deficiency anaemia which is microcytic. Macrocytic anaemia is unusual and when it does occur it is probably due to a deficiency of vitamin B_{12} or of folic acid. Folic acid levels are often low in rheumatoid arthritis, due to malabsorption.

Anaemia that is solely due to rheumatoid arthritis is seldom severe, the haemoglobin averaging around 11 g per 100 ml in women and 12 g per 100 ml in men. The rheumatoid anaemia results from a diminished number of circulating erythrocytes. There is only a slight reduction in Mean Corpuscular Haemoglobin Concentration (MCHC) to about 29–32 per cent (normal 30–36 per cent).

With iron deficiency, however, the MCHC is usually reduced to below 28 per cent, hypochromia is frequent and microcytosis the rule. In rheumatoid arthritis microcytosis suggests a concurrent iron deficiency. Table 1 below summarizes the characteristics of rheumatoid anaemia while Table 2 contrasts them with those of iron deficiency.

---

1. Characteristics of the anaemia of rheumatoid arthritis

- Normochromia.
- Normocytosis.
- Low serum iron – in inverse ratio with the sedimentation rate (normal: 50–100 mg per 100 ml – higher in males).
- MCHC 29–30 per cent (normal 32–36 per cent).
- Normal or reduced iron binding capacity.
- Rapid clearance of iron from plasma.
- Absent or poor therapeutic response to oral iron.

---

2. Difference between the anaemia of rheumatoid arthritis and iron deficiency

Rheumatoid arthritis	Iron deficiency anaemia
RBC and Hb reduced.	RBC and Hb reduced.
Serum iron binding capacity low or normal (normal: 250–400 mg per 100 ml).	Serum iron binding capacity raised.
Mean corpuscular haemoglobin concentration only slightly reduced.	Mean corpuscular haemoglobin concentration reduced.
Microcytosis rare.	Microcytosis the rule.

Mechanisms

Rheumatoid anaemia is largely due to excessive uptake of iron by the reticulo-endothelial (RE) system, which renders it unavailable for use in developing red cells.

The synovial tissues become heavily saturated with iron in the form of haemosiderin. Repeated injury to the inflamed joint may produce a succession of small haemarthroses followed by deposition of iron in the synovium. The lymph nodes in relation to inflamed joints become loaded with sequestrated iron.

In the bone marrow the red cells and their precursors are usually normal, though sometimes reduced in number. Haemosiderin deposits in the RE cells are usually increased. Reduction of sideroblasts in the presence of abundant stores of iron suggests that the RE system has an abnormal hunger for iron which ceases to be available for red cell formation.

Normally the body conserves iron, storing it for use as needed. It uses effete red cells as a source of iron for new haemoglobin. About 85 per cent of the iron from effete cells is rapidly returned to the circulation in new cells, the remainder being stored in the RE system. In rheumatoid arthritis it seems that re-utilization of iron from red blood cells is inefficient. Iron is stored as haemosiderin but it is not released normally. This failure of the RE system appears to be a direct result of the disease process and is proportional to the severity of the inflammation. Since the total body content of iron is about 4.5 g and since only about 1 mg is lost daily, there is an adequate amount of iron in an ordinary mixed diet. Pouring more iron into the body does not improve the anaemia but merely loads the system with unusable iron.

When iron deficiency exists in normal subjects, absorption of iron is increased, but it is diminished when the stores are replaced. Impaired absorption is not an important factor in the anaemia of rheumatoid arthritis. There is some haemodilution, with increase of plasma volume, but this again plays only a small part in causing anaemia.

Normal blood loss is about 0.5 ml a day. This may be considerably increased by treatment with salicylates and by bleeding into joints, but an average daily loss as high as 5 ml would be insufficient to cause anaemia even in a woman who was menstruating normally.

Management

Other things being equal, the anaemia of rheumatoid arthritis matches the activity of the disease. Effective treatment of the arthritis is also the effective treatment of the anaemia.

It was demonstrated several years ago that doses of corticosteroid or corticotrophin that suppress the joint disease also produce a dramatic rise in the serum and marrow iron, soon followed by a rising haemoglobin, even in the absence of iron supplements. Similar improvement occurs with any treatment that controls the inflammation. Although serum iron levels may be low, they rise when the inflammation subsides because the body has adequate iron stores already.

As for parenteral injections of iron it was found that they may raise haemoglobin initially but that this effect was short-lived with active rheumatoid disease and that repeated injections led to haemosiderosis and an exacerbation of joint pains. Iron injections are not a good form of long-term treatment because they may cause painful, even dangerous, reactions. Joint reactions sometimes follow intravenous iron injections even in nonrheumatoids.

In the presence of hypochromic and microcytic anaemia it is necessary to look for other diseases that may be causing blood loss: peptic ulcer – possibly drug-induced, piles and menorrhagia are obvious examples. If a macrocytic anaemia is discovered it must be investigated and treated in its own right. The anaemia is not part of the rheumatoid process and the most likely causes are B_{12} or folate deficiency.

FELTY'S SYNDROME

In 1924 Felty described five patients with rheumatoid arthritis and splenomegaly, three with brownish skin discoloration. Although most rheumatoid sufferers have lymphadenopathy and enlarged nodes which are palpable in relation to affected joints, these features are more obvious in Felty's syndrome as well as in Still's disease of children (see Chapter 11). More significantly, the neutrophil count is low, with increased risk of infections which may endanger life. Leg ulcers are common.

Four out of five patients improve with splenectomy, sometimes dramatically. Failures are often due to the existence of a splenunculus. In most patients the neutropenia improves rapidly after splenectomy, leg ulcers heal and infections are less frequent. Long-term follow-up, however, shows that the prognosis is not as good as it is in other rheumatoid patients. The efficacy of other treatment with agents such as lithium carbonate and testosterone is unproved.

SYSTEMIC LUPUS ERYTHEMATOSUS

Haematological changes are part of the disease. Anaemia is the rule and leucopenia and thrombocytopenia are both common. The anaemia is usually normochromic and normocytic but haemolytic anaemia occurs in 6–15 per cent of cases. A white-cell count below 4,000 per cu mm is present in about a fifth of cases and thrombocytopenia is to be found in 5–10 per cent. Lymphopenia is common. Neutrophils may be reduced. Very rarely, the bone marrow becomes hypoplastic. Leucocytosis may occur but is often the result of concurrent infection.

GOUT

The gouty patient is usually plump and florid. If anaemia is found, a search must be made for another cause. Gout may be secondary to certain blood disorders. It occurs in primary polycythaemia rubra vera and in cases of secondary polycythaemia. It may occur in acute or chronic leukaemia, malignant lymphoma, multiple myeloma, thalassaemia, sickle cell anaemia and the megaloblastic anaemia of tropical sprue.

In patients on anticoagulants reactions between warfarin and phenylbutazone or oxyphenbutazone may cause bleeding.

BLEEDING CAUSED BY ANTIRHEUMATIC DRUGS

Common minor effects

All the nonsteroidal anti-inflammatory agents (NSAIDs) may induce gastric erosion (see Chapter 29). Although this is unlikely to cause severe anaemia, melaena, haematemesis or insidious serious bleeding may occur with any of the NSAIDs, and particularly aspirin. Prepyloric ulceration and diffuse erosive gastritis may also occur. Patients who bleed with one NSAID often bleed with others.

Blood loss averages 3–5 ml a day on regular aspirin treatment, usually less on other NSAIDs. Some patients on aspirin may lose as much as 16 ml and suffer appreciable anaemia.

More serious complications

Aplastic anaemia from gold salts, d-penicillamine, the immunoregulatory agents (eg, azathioprine, cyclophosphamide), phenylbutazone and oxyphenbutazone.

Thrombocytopenia and resulting haemorrhage: as for aplastic anaemia above.

Haemolytic episodes from mefanemic acid and chloroquine.

Neutropenia from levimasole, gold, d-penicillamine, immunoregulatory agents and, very rarely, some of the NSAIDs.

Bleeding due to reactions with anticoagulants from phenylbutazone, oxyphenbutazone or, again rarely, other NSAIDs. All these are protein bound and may displace some substances as warfarin from serum proteins. Careful monitoring of the prothrombin time is essential.

Apart from phenylbutazone and oxyphenbutazone, blood dyscrasias are rare with the NSAIDs and much less common than they are with the long-term agents.

Antirheumatic drugs that can cause anaemia
- all NSAIDs
- gold salts
- d-penicillamine
- immunoregulatory agents
- mefenemic acid
- chloroquine
- levamisole
- phenylbutazone*
- oxyphenbutazone*

---

*Withdrawn in the UK

PRIMARY BLOOD DISORDERS

Just as some primary arthritic disorders can be associated with blood disorders so can some primary blood disorders be associated with arthritis.

Haemophilia

Haemorrhages into joints may cause acute swelling and discomfort resembling acute gout. It may lead to a type of osteoarthrosis, subsynovial changes leading to synovial hyperplasia and later capsular fibrosis with erosion of cartilage and subchondral bone cysts, sometimes with fibrous ankylosis. It used to be said that if a supposed haemophiliac could move all his joints by the time he was twenty-one years old, then the diagnosis must be wrong. While this may not entirely be true, joint changes are very common in haemophilia.

Acute leukaemia

There may be acute arthritis in one or a few joints and in children this may mimic rheumatic fever or Still's disease (see Chapter 11). This is particularly true in monocytic leukaemia where leukaemic infiltration occurs in and around joints.

Chronic leukaemia

This may rarely masquerade as an adult arthritis or gout in the knees.

Sickle cell disease

This may present in a child during a crisis as apparent acute rheumatic fever with diffuse polyarthritis – probably from marrow infarction adjacent to the bone. Aseptic necrosis of bone, often in the femoral head, may occur with destructive changes from thrombosis of the nutrient artery. This is usually associated with haemoglobin C disease. Salmonella osteomyelitis may also occur in the infarcted bones.

The disease is common in negro populations, whether in the form of homozygous sickle cell anaemia, a serious disease, or of heterogeneous sickle cell trait which is usually innocuous and not associated with anaemia, with only occasional symptoms. It is common in the negro population of Africa where about 30 per cent are affected, less common in the populations of Asia, the Middle East and the Mediterranean countries.

Diagnosis is made by haemoglobin electrophoresis and demonstration of sickling. In homozygous β thalassaemia (Cooley's or Mediterranean anaemia, thalassaemia major), which occurs most frequently in people of Mediterranean descent, anaemia starts in childhood with marked hepatosplenomegaly and bony abnormalities. But cases have been described in patients between five and thirty-three years with much pain, swelling and tenderness around the ankles.

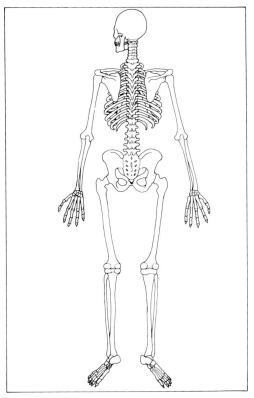

Figure 71 Sites most commonly affected in sickle cell disease; though it may occur anywhere.

PRACTICAL POINTS

● Blood disorders are often associated with rheumatic disorders.
● Always have a full blood count (FBC) carried out in chronic or unusual rheumatic disorders.
● Interpretation of a low haemoglobin level demands more than a blanket diagnosis of 'anaemia' and prescription of haemostatics.
● Clinical decisions have to be made as to whether the anaemia is part of the rheumatic process, whether it is due to a separate concurrent disease, or whether it is the result of the treatment being given.
● Remember that 'anaemia' is a sign that needs further investigation, and is not a final diagnosis on its own.
● Most rheumatic disorders are of unknown aetiology, and are treated in less than scientifically clear ways with drugs, which may relieve symptoms but which may cause unpleasant and dangerous side-effects on the blood.

24
Tuberculous arthritis

Tuberculosis is an old disease that has never been eradicated.

It is important to have this short chapter on tuberculous arthritis to remind readers that it has to be considered as a possible cause of an atypical arthritis with swelling, some pain and limitation of joint function. Unless recognized and treated effectively it can cause permanent disability and even death.

Tuberculosis is still a notifiable disease and has to be reported. The prognosis even now is less than perfect with some permanent joint damage in many cases.

PAST DECLINE

Tuberculosis remained common until a few years after the Second World War and many long-stay hospital beds used to be occupied by patients with pulmonary and surgical forms of this disease. Only a minority suffered from both forms because pulmonary tuberculosis was usually spread by inhalation from other human beings while most infections of the cervical glands and of bones and joints were acquired by drinking cow's milk. Numbers of new cases were falling before the war, but prevalence remained high.

Patients already debilitated by other chronic diseases were particularly likely to become infected with tuberculosis which had to be considered in the differential diagnosis of any low-grade febrile illness, any doubtful back pain or any disability confined to a single joint. It was not uncommon to find joint tuberculosis coexisting with some other form of chronic arthritis.

Effective antituberculous therapy came to Great Britain between 1946 and 1950 and it was soon realized that two or three drugs must be used concurrently to avoid bacterial resistance. In an early post-war (1946–7) study of ankylosing spondylitis, 7 of my first 100 patients, mostly young men from the Services, also had pulmonary tuberculosis. There was no tuberculosis among the next 100 cases and we have seen very little of it since. What had been the most common chronic infective condition in this country had faded into the background.

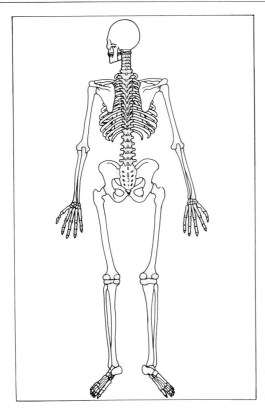

Figure 72   Sites more commonly affected by tuberculous disease of bone and joint; any segment of the spine may be affected.

PRESENT RESURGENCE

It had faded, but not for very long. In 1980 I attended a clinical morning in the English Midlands and it was entirely devoted to cases of bone and joint tuberculosis. Most of the patients came from India or Pakistan. For me, who had been a Tuberculosis Officer in London just before the war, it was like stepping back in time and I suddenly realized that few people in the audience had seen such cases before. In many, biopsy had produced a histological picture which seemed to confirm a clinical diagnosis of rheumatoid arthritis but tissue cultures were positive for tubercle bacilli. Most patients had involvement of only one or a few joints. Two recent papers reinforce the message that tuberculosis has completed its short vacation and is back at work.

1. From Manchester, England (Newton, Sharp and Barnes, 1981).[1] They describe 74 patients with nonspinal tuberculosis of bone and joint. Of these, 38 were first-generation immigrants, teenage males predominating. The greater trochanter was affected in 7, femur in 6, wrist in 6, hip in 11,

knee in 9, ankle and tarsus in 6 each, with other areas less common. A history of local trauma, often mild, was given in 16 cases, 14 of these having had injury to a joint or tendon sheath.

2. From London (Halsey, Reeback and Barnes, 1982).[2] They describe 58 cases of skeletal tuberculosis, 38 of which were immigrants. The spine was involved in 28 cases, other bones, joints or tendon sheaths in 30. A history of previous tuberculosis was present in 70 per cent of the indigenous and 31 per cent of the immigrant patients. The immigrants were younger than the indigenous patients and usually presented within five years of arrival in Britain. Of the 58, 6 had pulmonary tuberculosis (4 immigrant) and 4, all immigrant, had tuberculous adenitis. Of the 38 from overseas 33 came from the Indian subcontinent. The spine was involved in 28 patients (22 immigrant), the next most common sites being knee (5), ankle (5), hip (4), wrist (3) and ribs (3). Only 2 had tuberculous dactylitis.

Notification of tuberculosis in Great Britain fell from 12,300 in 1969 to 9,335 in 1979 but this was solely due to a fall in respiratory disease. Notification of nonrespiratory tuberculosis remained unaltered, being 2,372 in 1969 and 2,371 in 1979.

THE DISEASE ITSELF

Who gets it?

Bone and joint tuberculosis affects both sexes. It may occur at any age but is more common in children and the elderly and in the debilitated and malnourished. Patients taking corticosteroids are more susceptible to bacterial infection, including tuberculosis. The majority of cases in Great Britain are found in the Asian population.

Where in the body?

Some 3 per cent of tuberculous infections involve the locomotor system and half of these affect the spine. The dorsal spine is the most common site, followed by the knees, ankles, feet and sacro-iliac joints. Shoulders, elbows, wrists, fingers and pubes are less often affected. Bone or soft tissue may be involved. Infection is usually confined to one joint.

Clinical features

Onset is insidious, with swelling and restricted movement. Pain may be slight at first but increases with fatigue at the end of the day. Children may have muscle spasms at night ('night starts'). Fever is often present but may be slight.

There may be no physical signs at first and they are seldom as pronounced as those in other forms of arthritis. Early signs are swelling and tenderness with limitation of movement. The skin over the joint may be warm but it may also be cold and bluish red. Flexion deformities may develop and there may be tenosynovitis.

When the hip is involved there is usually a limp but little discomfort.

In spinal tuberculosis there are pains in the back or of girdle or root type, sometimes with an early angular kyphosis. The pains are eased by resting, by lying down and by support, while in ankylosing spondylitis the patient usually prefers to keep moving.

Tuberculosis of the sacro-iliac spine is usually unilateral. Ankylosing spondylitis commonly affects both sacro-iliacs.

Other tuberculous foci may be present in the lungs or cervical glands. A provisional diagnosis may be confirmed by X-rays or bacteriological examination.

Treatment

The main duty of the practitioner is to make the diagnosis early, before irreparable damage has been done.

Treatment of tuberculous arthritis is effective but has to be prolonged, perhaps for more than twelve months. It is based on:

1. **Chemotherapy** to eradicate infection.
2. **Rest** of the affected joints during the initial period of treatment by splintage or other means.
3. **Surgical excision** of infected areas (if infection persists), ie, synovectomy.
4. **Fixing the joint** (arthrodesis) or arthroplasty may be necessary if joint damage is severe.

PRACTICAL POINTS

● Don't forget the possibility of tuberculosis as a cause of a persistently swollen joint in an Asian immigrant.
● Don't forget the possibility of tuberculosis as a cause of persistent backache.
● Don't forget the possibility of tuberculosis in a limping child, affecting hip or knee.
● Joint tuberculosis is a general infection that requires general management.
● Unless diagnosis is early and treatment appropriate, permanent damage will result.

25

Endocrine disorders and arthritis

BACKGROUND

In an early (1873) description of myxoedema, Gull referred to the joint symptoms and the spade-like hands that he had found in some patients. But myxoedema is not the only endocrine disorder to show arthritic manifestations, which are sometimes the presenting features of the disease. Since most endocrine disorders are 'spot diagnoses' and since they are often easy to treat, it is important to bear them in mind when faced with a puzzling arthropathy.

HYPOTHYROIDISM

The fully developed clinical picture of hypothyroidism can be diagnosed from across the room or even over the telephone. The slow, low, grating speech, the coarse features, the yellowish dry skin – 'like a wax doll left in the shop window too long' – the falling hair, the scanty eyebrows and bare axillae, the slow pulse and the slow, pendulous reflexes, are all familiar.

Arthritic features

Any of the following may be found.

Carpal tunnel median nerve compression (see Chapter 15) with pains and numbness of the hands and wrists, tingling and discomfort radiating up to the shoulders, worse at night, with numbness and paraesthesiae over the thumb and first two and a half fingers on the radial side of the hand. This condition – usually but not always unilateral – occurs in up to half of patients with hypothyroidism, although often in a mild form.

Arthralgia and myalgia of shoulder and pelvic girdles.

Slight swelling, thickening and tenderness of joints, arthralgia and myalgia being more common than arthritis. Wrists, metacarpo- and metatarsophalangeals are more commonly affected than ankles and elbows. The proximal interphalangeal joints of fingers are occasionally involved. Effusions and synovial thickness with morning stiffness may simulate rheumatoid arthritis.

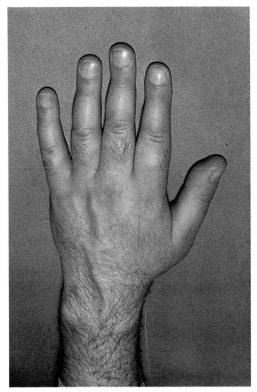

Figure 73   The hand in hypothyroidism.

True gout may occur rarely (see Chapter 12).

Treatment

Phenylbutazone may suppress thyroid function further, cause water loading and
aggravate the condition. Thyroxine should be started with small doses (0.05–0.1 mg
daily), to give the system time to adapt back to a normal state. In elderly and cardiac
patients angina or congestive heart failure may be precipitated by too rapid an increase
of dosage.

HYPERTHYROIDISM

This condition may coexist with rheumatoid arthritis but the relationship is obscure.
Loss of weight, tachycardia and muscle weakness are common to both conditions. In
hyperthyroidism myalgia is quite common, particularly in the shoulder girdle region,
often with fasciculation and muscle tenderness. But joint swelling is rare.

   In thyroid acropachy painless soft-tissue swelling of fingers and toes occurs, with

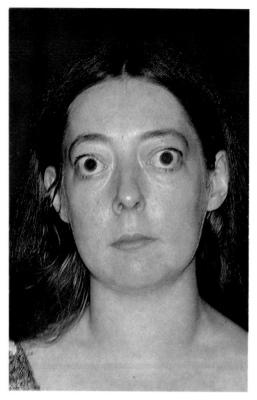

Figure 74   Typical features of hyper-thyroidism showing exophthalmos lid retraction, thyroid enlargement and smooth brow.

clubbing of the fingers, associated with exophthalmos (100 per cent) and pretibial myxoedema (80 per cent). These are patients who have been hyperthyroid and are now drifting into hypothyroidism after successful treatment. Serological tests for thyroid activity show that at the time when this condition develops only 10 per cent of the patients are still hyperthyroid, 50 per cent hypothyroid and the rest euthyroid. X-rays show irregular periosteal new bone formation involving the shafts of metacarpals, metatarsals and phalanges.

Treatment

Treatment is that of the thyroid state. The acropachy is not affected by treatment and remains unchanged.

HYPERPARATHYROIDISM

This condition is usually due to a parathyroid adenoma which produces excessive amounts of parathormone.

The accompanying symptoms are anorexia, constipation, weakness and lassitude while renal symptoms include polyuria, polydipsia and, occasionally, colic. Serum levels of calcium are raised (normal being 2.2–2.7 mmol/ml) as usually are those of alkaline phosphatase, while phosphate levels are diminished. Uric acid levels are raised in about half the cases. Serum urea levels rise at a later stage.

Arthritic features

X-rays show generalized osteoporosis with vertebral collapse and crush fractures, lytic cystic lesions, calcification of soft tissues and, occasionally, bony erosions resembling those of rheumatoid arthritis. Subperiosteal resorption over the phalanges gives a rough 'shark's tooth' appearance. Bone destruction may occur at later stages and is particularly troublesome if it affects the femoral heads.

The excessive amounts of parathormone may also cause the following arthropathies:

Synovitis, which most commonly affects the knees but may also be found in the hands, wrists, feet, ankles, elbows and spine, and is usually symmetrical. Joints may be tender, stiff and swollen – sometimes with effusion. The underlying lesion is softening and collapse of the subchondral bone.

Pyrophosphate arthropathy due to deposition of calcium pyrophosphate dihydrate (CPPD) in joint structures. This may produce acute pseudogout or a condition that resembles osteoarthrosis but shows linear calcification of the cartilages. The knees are most often affected.

A recurrent, low-grade polyarthritis is seen more rarely, with inflammatory episodes that may last several months. Pyrophosphate arthropathy may therefore resemble gout, osteoarthrosis or rheumatoid arthritis, but the serum calcium is raised in every case.

True gout Renal damage in hyperparathyroidism may cause diminished tubular secretion of uric acid leading to raised serum levels.

Treatment

The parathyroid adenoma must be removed, something which is often easier said than done. Tumours are multiple in about 10 per cent of cases and hyperparathyroidism is sometimes due to hyperplasia of the gland with no adenoma. Malignant tumours of the parathyroid are very rare.

HYPOPARATHYROIDISM

This condition causes pain and stiffness in the back and may be mistaken for ankylosing spondylitis. Other features are rashes, cataracts, fits and tetany. Trousseau's sign of carpopedal spasm may be produced by applying a tourniquet to the arm and Chvostek's sign of facial twitching, by tapping the facial nerve as it enters the cheek below the ear. Serum levels of calcium are low (normal being 2.2–2.7 mmol/ml), those of phosphate high. X-rays show calcification in ligaments and soft tissues and new bone

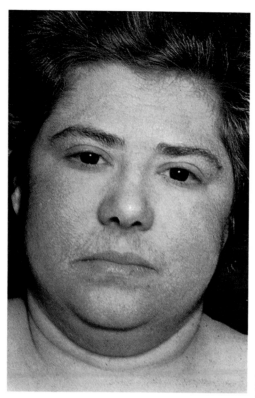

Figure 75 The typical puffy moon face of Cushing's syndrome, due in this case to an adrenal hyperplasia, with increase in fine hair growth and a plethoric appearance, even though the patient had a normal blood count.

formation round the pelvis and hips with increased bone density. Sacro-iliac joints remain normal.

CUSHING'S SYNDROME

This is due to hypersecretion of adrenal cortical hormones, particularly hydrocortisone (cortisol), by an adenoma or carcinoma of the adrenal cortex. But the same picture may be produced by medium or high dosage of any of the corticosteroid drugs that are prescribed for rheumatic disorders, or by the injection of corticotrophin or tetraco-sactrin. The patient becomes plump, moon-faced and somewhat plethoric but in contrast to this 'over-well' look, muscles are weak and may waste.

There is osteoporosis so that acute backache may be caused by vertebral crush-fractures, and ribs or long bones may be broken by minimal trauma. X-rays may show severe osteoporosis with intervertebral discs bulging to give a picture like that of cod-fish vertebrae.

When patients with rheumatoid arthritis are treated with corticosteroids or corticotrophin, reduction of the dose may lead to worsening of the suppressed disease which may also spread to joints that were previously unaffected, while raising the dose may lead to increased muscle weakness and discomfort. Reduction of medium or high dose corticosteroid therapy in nonrheumatic diseases is sometimes accompanied by tenderness and slight oedema of periarticular tissues but there is no true arthritis.

Whatever the condition for which corticosteroid therapy is used, reduction of dosage must be gradual because abrupt reduction may add the ill effects of adrenal insufficiency to exacerbation of the previously suppressed disease (see Chapter 30).

ACROMEGALY

This condition is due to excessive secretion of growth hormone by the pituitary. The cartilages are more vulnerable to degenerative change. Joint margins become calcified, ossified and hypertrophied, with prominent marginal osteophytosis, periarticular calcification and new bone formation at the insertions of tendons, capsules and ligaments. The affected joints become enlarged with thickened but ulcerated cartilages. Effusions may occur.

The commonest arthritic complaints are of carpal tunnel compression of the median nerve (see Chapter 15), backache and peripheral joint pains which affect the fingers and knees frequently, and the hips, ankles, shoulders, wrists and elbows occasionally. In the elbows crepitus is usually more impressive than discomfort. Affected joints may be abnormally mobile at first but they stiffen later. Hands and feet grow larger so that larger sizes of shoes and gloves are needed. The facial features are usually diagnostic.

Acute pseudogout from deposition of CPPD is a rare complication. Although the spine may stiffen and show gross radiological abnormalities it often remains mobile and may become excessively mobile as the intervertebral discs are thickened and hypertrophied.

The likely radiological findings in acromegaly are as follows:

1. Enlargement of the pituitary fossa (the most important finding).
2. Spine: wide disc spaces, anterior osteophytosis, bony bridging.
3. 'Tufting' of distal phalanges.
4. Enlarged joint spaces.
5. Bony outgrowths around joints.
6. Small areas of calcification in joint capsules and cartilages.
7. Thickened, widely spaced bony trabeculae.

Although the clinical and radiological changes in the spine may resemble those of ankylosing spondylitis, the sacro-iliac joints remain normal and this allows a distinction to be made.

Treatment

Treatment of acromegaly is directed to the pituitary. Hypophysectomy will often relieve the carpal tunnel symptoms but the other arthritic changes are irreversible, so

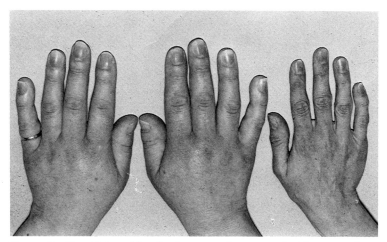

Figure 76 The thickened hands of acromegaly compared with a normal hand in a person of the same age.

treatment of joints is palliative. Fortunately the arthritic pains are seldom severe and only mild analgesics are needed.

Haemochromatosis

This is a hereditary disorder of iron metabolism, in which excessive amounts of iron are absorbed and deposited in the liver, pancreas and elsewhere, including the synovial membranes and the skin, giving rise to the name 'bronzed diabetes'. It is much more common in males than females in middle age, and is rare under the age of thirty. The mode of inheritance is unknown. The arthropathy is a noninflammatory degenerative process that begins in the small joints of the hands but goes on to affect the hips, knees and shoulders.

The first joint symptoms usually occur in the second and third metacarpophalangeal joints, where the patient notices twinges of pain on flexing his fingers. There is some bony swelling which may suggest osteoarthrosis, although the distribution of affected joints is more like that of rheumatoid arthritis.

Joint symptoms usually appear at the same time as other clinical manifestations but may occasionally precede or follow them. They occur in about half the cases of haemochromatosis and are usually mild, but some patients have a widespread joint involvement that affects the hip and other large joints. The hip is sometimes very painful and surgery may be needed. Acute or subacute attacks of CPPD arthritis (pseudogout) occur in a few cases, usually affecting the knees but sometimes affecting several joints to resemble rheumatoid arthritis.

Associated features which point to the true diagnosis are:

1. Skin pigmentation.
2. Loss of body hair.
3. Diminished sexual activity with testicular atrophy.
4. Hepatomegaly.
5. Glycosuria.

X-rays show joint narrowing with sclerosis of the margins and small bone cysts, 1–3 mm in diameter which are best seen in the bones adjacent to the metacarpophalangeal joints. Chondrocalcinosis may be present. Laboratory tests reveal a raised serum iron and evidence of diabetes mellitus. Liver biopsy shows iron deposition.

Treatment

Excess body iron must be removed by repeated venesection taking 500 ml of blood once or twice a week while maintaining the haemoglobin at 11 g per 100 ml and the haematocrit at or above 34 per cent. Since about 250 g of iron must be removed and 500 ml of blood contain 200–250 mg of iron, two to three years of frequent phlebotomy are usually needed. Desferrioxamine, a chelating agent, may be given parenterally but it is less effective than phlebotomy and more expensive.

Iron depletion does not improve existing arthropathy. The hope is to prevent further deterioration. NSAIDs are usually needed, with larger doses for acute episodes. Aspiration and intra-articular injection of steroid may be helpful in attacks of pseudogout. Surgery is sometimes needed.

The diabetes is treated in the usual way. Hepatic and/or cardiac failure may also have to be treated.

DIABETES MELLITUS

A number of arthropathies are associated with diabetes mellitus. They include the following:

Hypertrophic ankylosing hyperostosis (Forestier's disease)

This is a degenerative condition most marked in the dorsal and lumbar spine. It is characterized by formation of new bone appearing as bridges close to the anterior surfaces of the vertebrae with ossification of soft tissue including the longitudinal ligaments and the peripheral parts of the intervertebral discs. X-ray features are much more dramatic than clinical ones, there being no other symptoms than perhaps a mild backache.

It is said that up to half of patients with Forestier's disease have diabetes mellitus or at

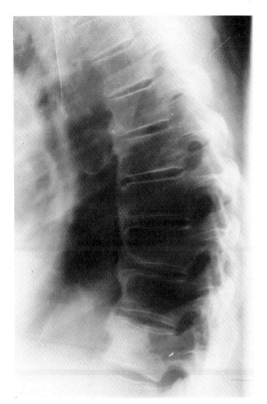

Figure 77 Hypertrophic ankylosing hyperostosis (Forestier's disease) showing anterior briding in dorso-lumbar spine different from the osteophytosis of the ageing osteoarthrotic spine where osteophytes project alongside disc protrusions and cause spur-like formations.

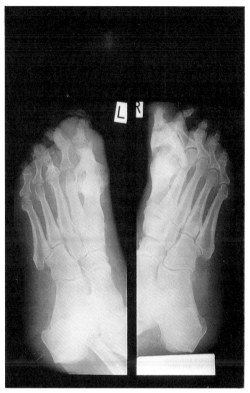

Figure 78 Destructive osteolytic changes in a diabetic in both big toes. The eroded infected proximal metatarsal on the right side suddenly appeared bathed in pus in an overlying ulcer on the sole of the foot and was extracted by the patient's wife, a qualified nursing sister, without pain as the patient had a diabetic neuropathy and could feel little.

least an impaired glucose tolerance but this is not my experience. After many years of running both diabetic and rheumatism clinics in the same hospital on different days, I estimate the association as around 10 per cent or less of diabetics having this condition which I usually found (by spinal X-rays) in obese patients who were past middle age.

Diabetic osteopathy

Diabetic osteopathy with osteolysis of the forefoot manifests itself by discomfort in the area with X-rays which show either a spotty or a generalized diminution of bone density of the distal ends of the metatarsals and the proximal parts of the adjacent phalanges. Pain is usually slight but occasionally severe.

The diabetes is sometimes mild or hitherto unrecognized. The lytic process may arrest itself or even show considerable improvement but it may proceed relentlessly to complete destruction of the bone ends.

Although neuropathic, infective and arterial disease may coexist with this condition there are many cases in which none of these factors are present and the cause of the osteolysis remains obscure.

Treatment is that of the diabetic state with symptomatic remedies for the local condition of the foot.

Diabetic pseudoscleroderma

Known also as 'the diabetic stiff-hand syndrome', this condition may occur early or late in the course of the disease.

In one of my patients, a man of forty-two with a diabetic mother, it developed three years before the advent of diabetes.

The hands become stiff rather than painful, with thickening of the skin of fingers and palms rather than the tight 'strangled' fingers of scleroderma. There is no apparent evidence of a diabetic neuropathy or arteriopathy, and pathological changes seem to lie in the periarticular collagen rather than in the joints themselves.

Other associated conditions

Dupuytren's contracture and periarthritis of the shoulder are more common in diabetics than in others, as is the peculiar thickening of collagen round the cervical spine which is known as scleroedema and gives the patient a thick bull-neck. It is clear that exclusion of diabetes mellitus is a diagnostic 'must' in any puzzling arthritis, periarthritis or connective tissue disorder.

'MENOPAUSAL ARTHRITIS'

This was a term applied in the 1920s in the United States to the disorder which Kellgren and Moore (Manchester 1952)[1] described as 'generalized osteoarthritis' (Chapter 10).

'Menopausal arthritis' is an unsatisfactory title because rheumatoid arthritis often begins at about the same time of life and the emotional or psychiatric disorders that afflict some menopausal women may intensify and exaggerate the symptoms of any arthropathy or other illness which happens to be present.

Since oestrogens favour a positive calcium balance and reduce bone resorption, their diminution at the menopause encourages the osteoporosis which may, thanks to immobility and disuse, afflict any disabled arthritic. Unfortunately there is no hard evidence that oestrogen therapy can prevent the mechanical fragility which is caused by osteoporosis and may lead to fractures, though it may lessen its progression. It is possible, however, that small doses of oestrogens may improve a variety of ill-defined aches and pains that are not accompanied by objective findings and are vaguely described as 'menopausal arthralgia'.

PRACTICAL POINTS

● The joints and connective tissues are often involved in endocrine disorders and they may be the first presenting features. This may confuse and delay diagnosis.
● **Hypothyroidism**   Note that the common carpal tunnel syndrome may be associated.
● **Hyperthyroidism**   Note pretibial myxoedema and finger clubbing as occasional associated features.
● **Hyperparathyroidism**   Gout and pseudogout may occur.
● **Hypoparathyroidism**   Associated with tetany and backache.
● **Cushing's syndrome**   Note osteoporosis and collapse of vertebrae.
● **Idiopathic haemochromatosis**   Joint symptoms in more than one half.
● **Diabetes**   Note ankylosing condition of dorsal and lumbar spine (Forestier's disease), osteolysis of forefoot, pseudoscleroderma, and Dupuytren's contracture.
● **'Menopausal arthritis'** is a vague and unhelpful label.

PART 5: MANAGEMENT AND THERAPY

26

When should you start and stop treatment?

BACKGROUND

Delay in starting treatment may prolong the patient's suffering, as in acute gout, or invite dangerous complications, as in giant cell arteritis.

Premature cessation of treatment will lead to a return of symptoms with a consequent drop in the patient's morale and his confidence in his physician. In rheumatoid and some other forms of arthritis it may allow a spread of the disease to joints that were previously unaffected.

GOUT

Treatment must be started at once. The patient who has had even one attack should be given a supply of an appropriate drug with instructions to start taking it as soon as another attack begins. Early dosage should be maximal and treatment should be tapered off rather than stopped suddenly. If symptoms recur during withdrawal it is necessary to resume a higher dosage. (See Chapter 12.)

POLYMYALGIA RHEUMATICA AND GIANT CELL ARTERITIS

These are probably different manifestations of a single disease (see Chapter 13). They may occur together or separately and the picture may change from one of polymyalgia to arteritis or vice versa. Treatment must be started as soon as a positive diagnosis is made. It must not wait on the result of arterial biopsy. If an artery is evidently inflamed, vision is already under threat and blind biopsy of an artery that does not seem to be inflamed may not yield a positive result.

But when should you stop treatment? The literature is usually vague about this and may recommend that therapy should be continued 'for several months or several years, exacerbations being common in the first two years.' In my experience of this disease it usually remains active for five years or even up to eight. I suggest that cautious withdrawal of dosage may begin after five years, with regular monitoring of the ESR and with instructions that the patient must resume higher dosage if there is any symptom of relapse.

RHEUMATOID ARTHRITIS

Treatment of rheumatoid arthritis is largely symptomatic (see Chapter 28). There is little strong evidence that the slow-acting drugs such as gold salts, penicillamine and the cytotoxic or immunoregulatory agents exert a deeper and more basic action on the course of the disease than the quick-acting NSAIDs. If there is adequate symptomatic control, the disease often abates or burns out as the months run into years; we have all seen this happen with both quick- and slow-acting drugs. However, rebound often occurs after discontinuation, within a few days with the former type of drug or within a few weeks with the latter.

In the Empire Rheumatism Council's double-blind, controlled multicentre trial of gold salts a significant therapeutic response was seen in the treated group but this improvement had disappeared one year after the completion of a six months' course of treatment.[1] Although great improvement and even complete remissions may occur on long-term treatment with gold salts, d-penicillamine, the antimalarials and the immunosuppressive or 'immunocorrective' drugs, recrudescence of disease activity may occur even years after stopping treatment. I have seen rheumatoid disease that appeared to have been completely suppressed but which flared up within three months of stopping treatment after five to six years of continuous therapy with gold salts and with d-penicillamine.

On present evidence it seems that the longer the effective symptomatic or suppressive treatment has been continued, the greater is the chance that the disease will have burned out under cover of the therapy; but there are few statistically significant data on this point and the natural history of rheumatoid arthritis is so variable and erratic that end results are impossible to foresee.

Provided that treatment is controlling symptoms, is well tolerated and has proved not to be toxic to the patient, it seems best, as with polymyalgia rheumatica (above), to maintain it at the lowest effective dose and only reduce it gradually over many months or years.

Unlike polymyalgia, however, rheumatoid arthritis is a disease in which increasing a dosage that has been reduced is less effective in bringing symptoms rapidly back under control, particularly when slow-acting agents are used. If the disease does flare up it may be necessary to return to full dosage or, often, to change to new medication.

OSTEOARTHROSIS

Osteoarthrosis is a disease that has to be managed rather than treated (see Chapter 10). There is little evidence that any present form of drug therapy brings permanent improvement and it has even been claimed that by reducing pain and stiffness, the NSAIDs may encourage further irreversible damage to joints. The effect of physical and pharmacological treatment is judged by its symptomatic effect and started or stopped according to the patient's needs and progress.

Management includes advice about modification of activity at home and work, adaptation of house and furniture, reduction of obesity, use of aids to mobility and getting help from the Social Services. Surgery has an increasingly important place in the treatment of osteoarthrosis, especially when one weight-bearing joint is severely affected.

THE SERONEGATIVE ARTHROPATHIES

Here again the treatment is that of the patient's symptoms and is reduced and finally discontinued as improvement occurs, but what has been said above about the treatment of rheumatoid arthritis with gold and other long-term agents is true of psoriatic and other arthropathies. The essence of the treatment of ankylosing spondylitis is to control pain and maintain mobility. There is no need to give drugs if the patient is comfortable and mobile. If he finds that he does not need his nightly NSAID it can be discontinued.

PRACTICAL POINTS

- There are few specific cures in rheumatology.
- Symptom-relief and patient-support are the pillars of good care.

27

How to manage the acute painful crisis

BACKGROUND

The heavy burden of chronic arthritis has many components. They include stiffness, pain, swelling, weakness, anxiety, depression and the feeling of frustration when every movement is thwarted by inefficiency as well as pain. But there are some special painful crises that transcend the daily grinding discomfort. The doctor who knows how to help his patient over them will receive all the gratitude that he deserves – and more.

RHEUMATIC SYNDROMES THAT CAN CAUSE ACUTE PAIN

Acute gout

The agony of acute gout is due to acute inflammation caused by the deposition of crystals in joints and/or surrounding tissue, usually of the big toe but sometimes of the ankle, knee, wrist, hand or elbow (see Chapter 12).

Because the agony rarely lasts more than a few days if it is properly treated it seldom causes the depression and anxiety induced by the less severe but longer-lasting inflammation of rheumatoid arthritis.

The treatment is to give full doses of a chosen NSAID at the first sign of onset of an attack. The drugs most popular in treatment of acute gout are:

Indomethacin 50 mg bd or tds, by mouth after food, with 100 mg by mouth or suppository at bedtime. This gives a total dosage of 200–250 mg on the first day. It should be reduced gradually as the attack comes under control, and discontinued when the patient has been free or nearly free of symptoms for forty-eight hours.

Colchicine 1 mg by mouth initially, followed by 0.5 mg every hour for three doses and then by 0.5 mg every two or three hours until a total of 5–6 mg has been given, or the attack has subsided, or until (as is often the case) the patient has begun to suffer from diarrhoea and perhaps vomiting.

Many doctors think that this old favourite has outlived its usefulness now that so many other drugs are at least as effective and do not cause this unpleasant gastro-intestinal irritation. The claim that colchicine can be used as a diagnostic as well as a therapeutic tool is valid, in that few other forms of arthritis respond to it. However, modern diagnosis should not be based on such shaky evidence.

Colchicine can also be given by intravenous injection of 2–3 mg, initially followed, if necessary, by 1 mg every six hours to a total of 5 mg. I do not advise this potentially dangerous use of a toxic drug when there are so many better and safer alternatives.

Naproxen 750 mg by mouth followed by 250 mg every eight hours until the attack is controlled. Suppositories of 500 mg are also available.

Fenoprofen 600–900 mg followed by 600 mg every six hours with reduction of the doses as control is achieved.

Azapropazone 600 mg followed by 600 mg after six hours and then by 300 mg every six hours, reducing as above: ie, around 2.4 g in the first twenty-four hours, then 1.8 g, then 1.2 g daily until symptoms have resolved.

Most of the other NSAIDs have been used and found effective in full doses. It happens rarely that NSAIDs fail to control an acute attack, usually because treatment has been delayed for several days. In such cases use either:

Corticotrophin 60–80 iu by im injection on the first day, reducing by 10 iu on each subsequent day, or:

Tetracosactrin 0.6 mg on first day reducing by 0.1 mg every one to two days, or, in very resistant cases, 0.75–1 mg, then halving dosage on day two and reducing by 0.1 mg every one or two days over a further seven to eight days. Discontinue the drug when the patient has been symptom-free for two to three days.

Pseudogout

In conditions due to acute deposition of crystals, such as pseudogout (see Chapter 12) from deposition of calcium pyrophosphate dihydrate (CPPD), the joint should first be aspirated to clinch the diagnosis and the attack usually subsides after complete aspiration (see Chapter 31).

The knee is the joint most commonly affected. Intra-articular corticosteroid injection may speed recovery. If this does not suffice, treat with an NSAID as in true gout. Colchicine is said not to be very effective.

Calcium hydroxyapatite crystals may cause a similar condition but they can only be identified by scanning-electron microscopy. Treatment is as for CPPD pseudogout. In the past, some corticosteroid preparations that were injected into joints caused a crystalline pseudogout syndrome.

Acute Reiter's (Brodie's) disease

This polyarthritis is more common in feet, ankles and knees than in hands, wrists and elbows (see Chapter 5). It may be almost as painful as acute gout and in very severe cases a similar dosage of corticotrophin or tetracosactrin may be needed for seven to ten days, with an NSAID being added as the intramuscular dosage is reduced after the first forty-eight hours. Oral analgesics may also be needed (see Table below) but this is not a condition for which I would use a potentially addictive drug.

I prefer corticotrophin or tetracosactrin to oral corticosteroids because courses of injections are more easily withdrawn and less likely to run on into prolonged treatment and the inevitable steroid side-effects (see Chapter 30).

Analgesics
- **Simple oral preparations**
    - aspirin or aspirin compounds
    - paracetamol or paracetamol compounds
    - codeine or codeine compound tablets
    - dextropropoxyphene or compound tablets
    - pentazocine
    - dihydrocodeine or dihydrocodeine compound tablets
    - nefopam
    - diflunisal
    - ethoheptazine compounds
    - meptazinol
    - suprofen
- **Stronger analgesics**
    - pentazocine by im or sc injection
    - buprenorphine by im or sc injection or sublingually
    - dihydrocodeine by im injection*
    - dipipanone and cyclizine by mouth (Diconal)*
    - nefopam by im or iv injection
    - morphine controlled release by mouth (MST 1 Continus)*

---

*Potentially dangerous and addictive. Subject to misuse of drugs legislation in many countries.

Severe acute discogenic backache

Someone in severe pain with a prolapsed disc, especially with sciatic radiation, should be kept in bed and given potent analgesics.

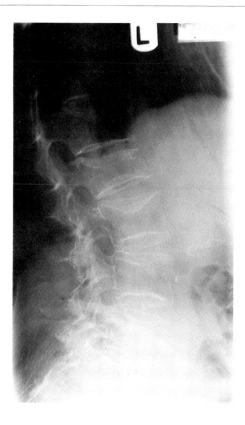

Figure 79 Osteoporosis of the lumbar spine with wedging and partial crushing of the vertebrae. Quite severe pain may occur for several weeks or months after such crush fractures.

Any of the stronger drugs in the Table opposite may be used two or three times a day during the first two or three days, but Diconal and dihydrocodeine injections should be withdrawn as soon as possible, with substitution of a milder oral drug. Early full analgesia often leads to rapid control with a shorter total period during which strong drugs have to be used.

The osteoporotic crush fracture

This usually occurs in older patients. If pain is severe, the treatment is the same as for discogenic backache (above). Mobilization should begin as soon as symptoms have settled sufficiently.

Acute bone pain from malignant disease

This may be due to metastases, myeloma or sarcoma of bone. Pain is not always intense but its effect is often magnified by anxiety and fear. If these can be allayed, simple analgesics or NSAIDs may suffice because the fact that pain is responding to what is known to be an antirheumatic drug will itself bring reassurance.

In more severe cases any of the stronger analgesics, including morphine or heroin, may be given by injection but preparations such as buprenorphine sublingually or Diconal or levorphanol orally may be preferred.

The dying patient   Where severe pain recurs constantly in a dying patient it is wise to give an oral preparation three to six hourly in Syrup BP in order to anticipate the pain and prevent its return. Each dose should contain 5–15 mg of morphine or diamorphine with alcohol. If there is nausea, vomiting or agitation, chlorpromazine or perchlorperazine should be added. Chlorpromazine Elixir (BPC 1973) may be used instead of Syrup BP in such cases. Levorphanol is almost as effective by mouth as by injection but as with some other narcotics it should not be given with alcohol as it renders therapeutic results unpredictable and may oversedate.

Much of the distress suffered by dying patients is not simply due to pain but to a mixture of causes which include fear, anxiety and nausea. An analgesic that does not allay other causes of distress, or even aggravates them, will do more harm than good and should be changed. Good nursing and the concern of the doctor are often as comforting as analgesics or other drugs and can never fail to enhance their beneficial effects.

Terminally ill patients with rheumatoid disease

If pain is severe and the outlook hopeless, treat as for the dying patient (above).

Injury

Injuries may cause severe pain to arthritics who are particularly liable to strains, subluxations, torn muscles and fractures. Osteoarthrotic knees often swell as a result of injury or excessive use and any rheumatic joint is especially prone to harm. Fractures are more common in rheumatoid patients due to osteoporosis, and in ankylosed spondylitics because of bone rigidity.

Treatment of bony injury lies in the hands of the orthopaedic or neurosurgeon, but damage to soft tissues can be greatly relieved by rest, support, local applications, analgesics and injections of lignocaine, corticosteroids or, in some cases, both.

Atlanto-axial subluxation may occur in rheumatoid arthritis and, rarely, in ankylosing spondylitis. If it is accompanied by neurological signs of pressure it calls for neurosurgical attention. The most common symptom suggesting this subluxation in rheumatoid arthritis is pain radiating into the occiput with paraesthesiae in shoulders and arms on moving the head. Radiography will show undue mobility with more than 3 mm separation between the odontoid peg and the axial arch when the neck is flexed. Surgery is only necessary in a small minority of those who are without symptoms of compression of the cord.

Sepsis

Sepsis in or adjacent to a joint may cause acute pain, fever and general malaise. Aspiration (see Chapter 31), drainage and appropriate medication are indicated as necessary.

Bursitis

This is seldom very painful unless the bursa is septic or tensely distended with fluid or viscous material. Surgical drainage is then necessary if aspiration proves inadequate. Bursae that may be affected are the subacromial, those of the knee, the iliopsoas and, rarely, the olecranon. Ischial or ischiogluteal bursitis may cause irritation of the sciatic or the posterior femoral cutaneous nerve. In such cases palpation of the ischial tuberosity usually causes considerable discomfort. In most cases the pain of bursitis is less severe and can be adequately dealt with by an injection of a corticosteroid and/or a local anaesthetic. A septic bursa must be treated like any other abscess.

PRACTICAL POINTS

- **Acute gout** Control with NSAIDs.
- **Pseudogout** Control by aspiration of affected joint.
- **Acute Reiter's disease** Control by corticotrophin or tetracosactrin if NSAIDs are inadequate.
- **Acute discogenic backache** Use strong analgesics.
- **Malignant bone disease** Use opiates or other strong analgesics.
- **Terminal rheumatoid arthritis** Control with strong analgesics.
- **Acute bursitis, unless septic, aspirate and inject corticosteroid.**

28

How to manage
rheumatoid arthritis

BACKGROUND

Were I to be given one wish which would be granted by a therapeutic fairy queen, rheumatoid arthritis would be the single disease that I should most like to see eradicated. Although it affects only 1–2 per cent of the population, much less than spinal degenerative disorders and osteoarthrosis of other joints, it has a much more serious effect on general health and morale, lasts longer and is more crippling (see Chapter 10). It is an erosive condition, destroying bone and cartilage by an inflammatory process that almost rivals malignancy in its capacity to eat up tissues. It causes fever, loss of weight and systemic upset, and throws a greater strain on the spirit than most diseases. In all these ways it resembles a chronic infective condition such as tuberculosis. Although it does not have the lethal effect of that disease it certainly shortens life in chronic progressive cases and can even prove fatal within quite a few years in Felty's syndrome or where vasculitis or other extra-articular complications are present.

Quite apart from its effect on expectation of life, rheumatoid arthritis probably causes the longest-lasting pain that any patient is called upon to endure while also suffering from systemic illness, anxiety and depression. As one patient said to me: 'Life is a long grey tunnel stretching ahead of me. When I wake up and pains and stiffness are no better than they have been for two years past, the future seems to hold nothing for me.'

MANAGEMENT PRINCIPLES

The management of any arthritic patient is an individual problem in every case. Even if two people have much the same severity of the same disease in the same joints they cannot be expected to react to it in exactly the same way. Rheumatoid arthritis is no exception.

What can the doctor do to help in the control of this very unpleasant disease? In view of the long period of illness which lies ahead, it is necessary to instruct the patient, and those who are close to him, in the art of living with the disease and, hopefully, on top of it. This is a condition that must be managed rather than treated.

Information

If the patient does not get adequate information from his doctor he will probably turn to friends, relatives, the lay press and other unreliable sources, which, for all their good intentions, may mislead him by giving advice about conditions from which he does not suffer.

The practitioner should tell the patient the diagnosis and inform him about the natural history of his disease. Even though the prospect is gloomy, the known is easier to face than the unknown and it may be possible to reassure him that he will not suffer all the complications that he has seen afflicting a relative or friend.

Organizations listed in the Useful Addresses section will be able to help him with a choice of booklets and put him in touch with self-help groups.

Rest and exercise

When managing any case of rheumatoid arthritis it is essential to adjust the balance between rest and activity, between attempting too much and being content with too little. The patient who tries to do too much at a time when the disease is very active may suffer an exacerbation that will continue for weeks or months or even lead to irreversible deterioration, but the patient who rests too much may develop fixed deformities, usually in flexion.

Rest programmes and exercise are discussed in Chapter 32. The patient must be given detailed and exact instruction about what exercise and exercises should be attempted and regularly performed in his particular case and at each particular stage of his illness. He must also be told what periods of rest are to be taken and what supports or splints are to be worn, when and for how long.

All joints must be put through the fullest possible range of movements every morning and evening. This can often be done more easily and effectively after a hot bath or shower or after warming by a fire or lamp. There is no special virtue in any particular form of heat but a greater range of movement can often be achieved when a joint is actually immersed in warm water.

Patients with rheumatoid arthritis are often at their worst during the night hours and in the early morning when they wake too soon. The hours and quality of sleep at night and the time spent in bed must therefore be discussed and short periods of rest in midmorning or afternoon may be advised, especially if inflammatory features of active arthritis are present.

Home physiotherapy

Apart from exercises, this includes hot-water soaks and other forms of heat. Ice packs may bring some relief to swollen stiff joints.

Modification of working and living conditions

A great deal of help is available but the responsibility for providing it is divided between a variety of statutory and voluntary bodies whose duties overlap to a bewildering extent. The occupational therapist and the medical social worker are best qualified to advise the patient and her doctor about what needs to be done and how to get it done.

General domestic advice

Advice about clothing, bedding, travelling, diet and domestic and marital activities should be given. A duvet, for example, is often easier to manage than bed clothing; and zips are simpler than buttons. The occupational therapist can advise about gadgets which have been devised to facilitate dressing and eating. (See Chapter 33 for dietary recommendations.)

Medicines

Drug treatment should be kept to the lowest completely effective dosage and the patient should be thoroughly instructed about what to expect from the medicines he is taking, when to take them, when to vary the dose, what unwanted effects to recognize and how, if possible, to avoid them. He should not be given a long and comprehensive list of all possible unwanted effects, many of which he might then experience within a short time of receiving the information, but he should be alerted to the possibility of the ones most likely to occur with his particular medication. The possibility of such reactions should be appreciated but their advent not anticipated. The action of steroidal and nonsteroidal anti-inflammatory drugs and analgesics should be explained to the patient who is to take them and he should have some knowledge of their therapeutic and toxic action. I am still amazed by the number of intelligent patients who are unable to give the name of the drug they have been taking for months or even years.

Many patients are diffident about reporting harmful effects but they must be encouraged to do so. The treatment of rheumatoid arthritis often involves pushing the dose of potentially harmful drugs to the limit of tolerance (see below).

Home visits

Visits by home nurses and helps must be arranged. Professional physiotherapy is sometimes provided at home by State-run health services.

THE PRACTITIONER'S ROLES

The management of rheumatoid arthritis (or severe osteoarthrosis) is a team affair, the team being the patient's practitioner, the rheumatologist, physio- and occupational therapists, nurse, social worker, chiropodist and specialists as required. The practitioner, as captain of the team, must be in close contact with the other members and closest of all to the patient. Without close rapport the whole scheme of management disintegrates. For this reason constant changes of medical attendant and team members is highly undesirable; continuity of management programme and team membership is essential.

The practitioner knows that rheumatoid arthritis is often if not usually a life sentence for his patient and that the care of each rheumatoid sufferer is a life sentence for himself. The patient needs to be seen at least once a month, even if this must continue for over twenty years. He ought to be referred to a specialist because only a specialist sees enough patients to be able to know what treatment now seems to offer most hope. The practitioner should not shrink from repeated referral for a disease whose treatment ought to be aggressive and is still the subject of continuing reassessment. He is usually the person best qualified to decide that a period of in-patient treatment is necessary and there are times when he may want to suggest that a different sort of specialist, an orthopaedic surgeon, perhaps, or a psychiatrist, should be called into consultation.

FIRST-LINE DRUGS

If drugs do not cure they can at least help the patient to adopt an enthusiastic attitude towards his condition, rather than one of resignation.

The first line of drug treatment for active rheumatoid arthritis is the regular administration of an NSAID (see Chapter 29). If the condition responds to such a drug, with the help of appropriate rest and activity, treatment can be continued. If it has failed to respond at the end of three to six months and especially if the patient's condition is worsening in spite of full dosage and adequate co-operation, it is necessary to consider the use of second-line drugs.[1]

SECOND-LINE DRUGS

Gold salts

The only preparation now available in Great Britain is sodium aurothiomalate, which has now been used in the treatment of rheumatoid arthritis for some fifty years. How it works is still obscure but it has been shown to reduce the inflammatory component very slowly and gradually. Whether it reduces or halts erosive changes in bones remains doubtful. The therapeutic effects may take up to three months to manifest themselves and they then usually continue so long as therapy is maintained, but when treatment is stopped, symptoms and signs of the disease return slowly in most cases. They have been known to return a few weeks or months after treatment was stopped in cases that had seemed to be under control for as long as five years and for that reason most doctors continue treatment at a lower dosage for several years at least.

Dosage   Begin with two test doses of 0.1 mg and 0.25 mg given at a week's interval, intramuscularly. If there is no ill effect, give 50 mg weekly until the rheumatoid condition appears to be controlled. Then increase the interval between injections to two, three and eventually four weeks. An alternative is to reduce the dose to 20 mg and then 10 mg at weekly intervals, but full dosage at longer intervals is usually preferable.

Side-effects   Treatment must be carefully monitored because gold is potentially toxic. The most common ill effect is a rash which occurs in about 30 per cent of those treated, usually within the first six months. It is sometimes mild and transient but may take the form of a severe exfoliative dermatitis lasting many months. Although it may be possible to restart with smaller doses this is probably inadvisable because rashes often recur.

Gold injections may cause renal irritation with proteinuria or haematuria but occasionally with a nephrotic syndrome including oedema. This condition usually resolves on stopping the drug and seldom causes permanent damage, but gold treatment should not be resumed. The most dangerous complication of gold treatment is a blood dyscrasia and deaths have resulted from aplastic anaemia, from haemorrhage due to thrombocytopenia and, less commonly, from agranulocytosis. Uncomfortable buccal ulcers may occur without blood changes.

Possible side-effects of gold salts
- Mild rash
- Severe exfoliative dermatitis
- Renal irritation
- Blood dyscrasia
- Buccal ulcers

Monitoring   Because of their dangerous side-effects no physician should undertake long-term treatment with gold salts unless close monitoring is possible.

The urine must be tested every week and there must be full blood and platelet counts and estimations of the ESR every two weeks for the first three months and monthly thereafter, the blood examinations preferably being done a day or two after the last gold injection.

The patient should sign an initial consent form, as he would before an operation, and he should state that he understands the risks that are present and is willing to take them.

He should carry a card stating that he is on gold treatment and the physician should maintain it, showing the dose given on each date, the total cumulative dosage and preceding blood examination, with platelet count, white cell total and differential counts, ESR and any adverse findings such as rash, mouth ulcers or urinary abnormality. Blood figures should be listed quantitatively (see example below) so that any sudden change or insidious tendency may be clearly observable.

Date	Platelets	Hb	RBC	WBC	ESR	Urine
1.1.82	250,000	12.6G	5.2m	7,500 (N 4,000, L 2,500, E 350, B 150, M 500)	44 mm in 1 hour	NAD
15.1.82	280,000	12.0G	5.0m	7,600 (N 3,800, L 2,700, E 400, B 100, M 600)	40 mm in 1 hour	NAD
29.1.82	260,000	11.8G	4.7m	6,700 (N 4,400, L 1,600, E 100, B 100, M 500)	32 mm in 1 hour	NAD

It is particularly important that platelets should be counted. A laboratory report that 'platelets appear to be normal in number' is unreliable and often misleading and cannot be accepted in monitoring the condition of a patient who is receiving long-term treatment with gold or any other agent which may have an adverse effect on the blood.

D-penicillamine[2]

Dosage Smaller doses are now being given. An initial oral dosage of 125–250 mg daily should be slowly increased by 125 mg each month to a final maximum of 500–750 mg. If a larger daily dose is to be given in a resistant case the physician must be aware of the danger and proceed with increased caution. As with gold (above), improvement may not be seen for three to six months and, again as with gold, it is wise to continue treatment for several years although possibly with a dose reduced to 250–500 mg daily.

Side-effects Yet again, as with gold, the most important complications are blood changes and renal toxicity. The same careful supervision is therefore necessary, with urine checks, and blood and platelet counts. Other untoward effects include loss of taste, which is usually transient even when dosage is maintained. Rashes may occur early or late in treatment. If early they may be transient and treatment can be resumed after an interruption, but rashes that first appear after ten to twelve months are more serious and indicate that treatment must be stopped. Rarer toxic reactions include a syndrome that resembles myasthenia, one that resembles systemic lupus erythematosus and another that resembles pemphigus.

The antimalarials

Chloroquine and hydroxychloroquine were thought to be dangerous to use because of their threat to vision but when doses were reduced retinal toxicity became rare. It is now usual to give 200–250 mg of chloroquine or 400 mg of hydroxychloroquine daily and dosage can often become intermittent after the first year. Ophthalmic examination must be carried out before treatment is started and then repeated every three months. It must include definition of visual fields using red and white light. In other respects the antimalarials are less toxic than gold salts or penicillamine.

Immunoregulatory agents

With levimasole, azothioprine and other immunoregulatory agents, very careful monitoring is needed, and they are probably best controlled from special clinics and rheumatism units.

Corticosteroids

These are more fully discussed in Chapter 30. At small doses of under 7 mg prednisolone or the equivalent of some other preparation they are usually well tolerated but it was the treatment with higher doses that earned them the reputation of miracle drugs in the early days and their bad reputation for toxicity soon afterwards. In daily doses of 7 mg or less they may ease the morning stiffness and other symptoms of rheumatoid arthritis. Short booster courses at higher doses are often effective but they cannot always be reduced without a return of symptoms.

The phase of dramatic response to high dosage was sometimes described as 'the honeymoon period' and that of returning symptoms on dose reduction was called 'the matrimonial period'. Unfortunately the use of high doses caused some deaths. Nevertheless, if the corticosteroids are used with discretion and at conservative dosage they are the most effective anti-inflammatory agents at our disposal, even if their main uses are in disorders other than rheumatoid arthritis.

Corticotrophin and tetracosactrin, also effective agents given intramuscularly, have a useful but limited part to play in the management of this disease, usually to cover acute exacerbations that are being treated in hospital.

Other drugs

Antidepressants, anxiolytics and analgesics all have their part to play in the treatment of rheumatoid arthritis (see Chapter 27). It may be necessary to treat dyspepsia, often induced or aggravated by drugs (see Chapter 21).

PRACTICAL POINTS

- Rheumatoid disease affects the whole patient and not only the joints.
- Course is unpredictable. Only a minority become severely crippled.
- There are no cures but much can be achieved by good management, drugs and support.
- Management of a patient with rheumatoid arthritis – or any other chronic arthropathy – involves:
  1. Some education in the understanding of the natural history of his particular disease and the general principles underlying its management.
  2. The correct ratio of rest – local and general – to exercise; exercises; and the use of splints and physical therapy.
  3. Diet and weight control.
  4. Use of Social Services.
  5. Use of drugs and their monitoring.
  6. Attendance at surgery, clinic or special centre.
  7. Hospital admission when necessary.
  8. Surgery in selected cases.

29

Which nonsteroidal anti-inflammatory drug?

BACKGROUND

During the latter half of the nineteenth century German chemists gave the world its first useful drugs for the treatment of arthritic disorders: phenacetin, amidopyrine (aminopyrine), acetyl salicylic acid (aspirin) and paracetamol (acetaminophen) eased pain and fever and were introduced as antipyretic analgesic agents. The first two, along with some others, have now been withdrawn because of toxicity but aspirin and paracetamol are still popular and both are available without prescription.

Aspirin and paracetamol

Both aspirin and paracetamol are excellent drugs for relieving pain and reducing fever. For simple pain relief in any condition that is likely to subside spontaneously in a few hours or days they can be taken as found necessary. Aspirin in high doses (over 4 g daily) can be seen to reduce inflammatory changes in rheumatoid arthritis. Paracetamol in doses up to 6 g daily does not have this effect[1] although it is reported to reduce inflammation in some other conditions such as peri-odontal swelling after dental extraction.[2]

WHAT NSAIDs ARE AVAILABLE?

Aspirin (1899) was the first of the NSAIDs and is still in general use. The second was phenylbutazone (1952), followed by its metabolite, oxyphenbutazone (1956), and indomethacin (1964). Since then a large number of nonsteroidal agents have been introduced (see Table overleaf) but their availability varies from one country to another, mainly because of local laws and regulations.

THE EFFECTS OF NSAIDs

All NSAIDs share the three properties in varying degrees:

  1. Anti-inflammatory.
  2. Analgesic.
  3. Antipyretic.

NSAIDs

—aspirin and other salicylates
—benorylate
—diflunisal
—salsalate
—choline magnesium trisalicylate
—aloxiprin
—azapropazone
—mefenamic acid
—flufenamic acid
—indomethacin
—sulindac
—tolmetin
—ibuprofen
—ketoprofen
—fenoprofen
—naproxen
—flurbiprofen
—tiaprofenic acid
—fenbufen
—diclofenac
—piroxicam

None is as effective as the corticosteroids in reducing inflammation but they do not have the unwanted endocrine effects that are repeatedly seen during medium or high dosage with corticosteroids (see Chapter 30). Their essential action, like that of the steroids, is upon the peripheral tissues, while that of the simple analgesics is mainly upon the central nervous system, although aspirin has both peripheral and central effects.

The NSAIDs are often described as 'antirheumatic', although they are not, in the strict sense, curative. Their effect is to make the patient's life more comfortable by suppressing the inflammatory features of his disease. It is possible, even probable, that this dampening of the inflammatory fires contributes to their eventual extinction, but it remains unproved.

Side-effects of NSAIDs

While not sharing the unwanted effects of the corticosteroids, the NSAIDs bring troubles of their own. The most common of these are gastro-intestinal; any NSAID may cause them although some do it more often than others. Less usual ill-effects are skin rashes, depression of kidney function, hepatic toxicity, tinnitus and deafness, and allergic phenomena including asthma and mucocutaneous reactions. According to present clinical and pharmacological evidence about the NSAIDs:

1. Gastric or gastroduodenal irritation is most likely to be caused by aspirin, followed, in uncertain order, by indomethacin, tolectin, flurbiprofen, fenoprofen and high dosage of naproxen. Different studies give different figures (see Chapter 21). The least likely to cause it seem to be diflunisal and sulindac,[3] fenbufen,[4] and, except at high doses, ibuprofen.[5]

2. Diarrhoea is associated with anthranilates (mefenamic and flufenamic acids) in 10 per cent of cases in which they are used.[6]

3. Skin rashes were frequent during the use of alclofenac and led to its withdrawal from the market.

4. Light sensitivity was common with and peculiar to the use of benoxaprofen. Onycholysis (separation of nails from their beds) was not uncommon with this drug, but led to little inconvenience and was painless. The drug has now been withdrawn.

5. Deafness and tinnitus are most common with aspirin; headache and 'muzziness' or dizziness with aspirin or indomethacin.

6. Blood dyscrasias have been reported, rarely, with almost all the NSAIDs, but only often enough to cause concern with phenylbutazone and oxyphenbutazone, now withdrawn in Great Britain.

7. Aspirin allergy is seen in two forms, that of bronchospasm ('aspirin asthma') and that of urticaria and angioneurotic oedema. Both forms are due to prostaglandin inhibition and can be caused by aspirin or almost any other NSAID, although not by paracetamol, sodium salicylate or dextropropoxyphene. Quite small doses such as 30 mg of aspirin or 5 mg of indomethacin can cause a serious or even a fatal reaction. A history of aspirin allergy is therefore a warning of possible trouble with another NSAID. Skin tests are negative and of no value as a means of predicting this allergy.

8. Oedema of ankles may result from depressed renal function but is more often due to the arthritis itself, or to enforced immobility or to unrelated cardiac or renal disease.

9. An occasional 'toxic reaction' may be due to chance. Every placebo group in every drug trial shows its scatter of common 'reactions', including rashes, indigestion and, rarely, even blood changes. Great care has to be taken when assessing adverse effects. A wide mesh catches too few fish and a small mesh catches too many. Two drugs, alcohol and nicotine, which are widely used but seldom considered by patients, may affect the picture, while other drugs taken for other disorders may alter, potentiate or diminish the effect of the antirheumatic drug.

INTERACTIONS WITH NSAIDs

As people age, their kidneys, liver and other organs become less capable of metabolizing and/or excreting drugs and their metabolites. Since many, especially those in the older age groups, are now receiving several drugs at the same time and since these drugs may react with one another, it is worth considering the potential interactions of the more common NSAIDs given for rheumatism with those used for cardiac, thrombo-embolic and some other disorders.

Aspirin

Para-aminosalicylic acid (PAS) is given for pulmonary tuberculosis. It raises the blood level of salicylate and increases the risk of salicylism. This danger is greater with large doses of PAS.

Ammonium chloride diminishes urinary clearance and leads to increased plasma salicylate but the increase is unlikely to be great or to cause symptoms.

Ascorbic acid has an effect similar to that of ammonium chloride above.

Antacids increase urinary clearance and may cause a drop in plasma salicylate levels but this effect is unlikely to be noticed clinically.

Alcohol increases the tendency of salicylates to cause gastro-intestinal irritation and gastric haemorrhage.

Heparin and oral anticoagulants (eg, warfarin). If aspirin is taken with any of these agents there is an increased risk of haemorrhage.

Antidiabetic drugs (eg, the sulphonylureas). Aspirin potentiates their effect with added risk of hypoglycaemia.

Methotrexate   The clinical effect is increased by aspirin, which displaces it from plasmic proteins.

Drugs for gout   The uricosuric action of probenecid, sulphinpyrazone and phenylbutazone is inhibited by aspirin, even in small doses. There may be an increase in serum uric acid and an attack of gout may be precipitated.

Corticosteroids   If long-term therapy is withdrawn without reduction of concurrent aspirin dosage there may be symptoms of salicylism.

Spironolactone   Aspirin may inhibit sodium excretion but serious trouble is unlikely.

Imipramine and nortriptyline   Aspirin may increase serum levels and side-effects but these are seldom troublesome.

Warfarin Bleeding may be severe. To maintain correct prothrombin times when phenylbutazone is given concurrently it may be necessary to reduce the dose of warfarin by 50–75 per cent.

Antidiabetic drugs (eg, tolbutamide, chlorpropamide, acetohexamide, tolbutamide). Hypoglycaemia may be profound.

Phenytoin Any of its side-effects may occur more readily.

Diuretics and antihypertensives Phenylbutazone may reduce their effect and cause salt and water retention.

Cholestyramine This anion-exchange resin may cause reduced absorption of phenyl-butazone.

Thyroid conditions Phenylbutazone may cause subthyroidism and interfere with the interpretation of thyroid function tests.

Other NSAIDs

Azapropazone is chemically related to phenylbutazone and may also potentiate the action of warfarin.

Indomethacin reduces the action of frusemide, the thiazide diuretics and propranolol. Its own therapeutic effect is increased if probenecid is given concurrently. On present evidence this combination brings little or no increase of unwanted effects.

Tolmetin is highly bound to plasma proteins. There is, to date, little evidence of toxic interaction with other protein-bound drugs but the possibility must be borne in mind.

Diclofenac is 99 per cent protein bound. High levels of aspirin or phenylbutazone may diminish the degree of bonding and reduce bio-availability.

All NSAIDs

Every NSAID may displace drugs from protein-binding sites.

Warfarin   In all patients receiving warfarin with an NSAID it is necessary to observe prothrombin times with special care, in spite of reports that warfarin has been given safely with indomethacin, tolmetin and several of the propionic agents. The lower level of protein binding exhibited by indomethacin, compared to phenylbutazone, probably explains the reported difference in interactions.

Antidiabetic drugs   Careful observation of the blood sugar is needed when any oral antidiabetic is to be given with any NSAID.

POTENCY OF NSAIDS

Which, then, are the most potent NSAIDs? There is great individual variation between patients and while one may react poorly to drug A and do well on drug B, another will behave in an exactly opposite way. Generally speaking, the first three on the market, aspirin in full doses, phenylbutazone and indomethacin, have not been surpassed, but aspirin may cause much gastro-intestinal upset and unpleasant cerebral effects, phenylbutazone carried a small but real risk of aplastic anaemia, and indomethacin may cause dyspepsia, though this is diminished by using it in suppository, delayed action or slow release forms (sodium indomethacin trihydrate in special capsule). Indomethacin may also cause various cerebral sensations, but this usually happens at high dosage and responds to reduction.

It has long been known that there are some patients who fail to respond to certain drugs. In a study by Baber and his colleagues,[7, 8] eight subjects known to be nonreactors to indomethacin were reintroduced into a drug trial, the nonreactors being unknown to the assessors. The same eight patients again failed to respond to indomethacin although they, like the assessors, did not know what drug was being given. Blood levels were the same in reactors and nonreactors, showing that the difference was not due to a failure of absorption. It seems that these eight patients failed to benefit from the drug because their bodies were handling it in a biologically different way. As Huskisson noted[9] in reporting a comparison of four chemically related (propionic) agents, there is more interpatient than interdrug variation in clinical response.

PATIENT PREFERENCE

A patient may prefer a particular drug because:
1. It works better for him and eases his symptoms more effectively.
2. It is less toxic for him.
3. He 'feels better on it.' This is often his way of saying that he does not have the low-grade nausea, anorexia, looseness of bowel motions or cerebral sensations – the almost subclinical side-effects – that he may have experienced with other drugs.
4. It tastes better.

5. It need only be taken once or twice a day, which is more convenient.

The four most popular NSAIDs in Great Britain today are:

- **Indomethacin**, which is very effective and popular, in spite of side-effects.
- **Piroxicam**, which is effective, relatively nontoxic and need only be taken once a day.
- **Naproxen**, which is effective, usually nontoxic and only has to be taken twice a day.
- **Ibuprofen**, which is well tolerated even if less potent.

DOCTOR CHOICE

Trial and error is the only certain way of finding out which NSAID is most suitable for a particular patient but before starting him on a new agent it is sensible to ask him the following questions:

1. What NSAIDs has he had previously and what was their effect?
2. What ill effects has he had with other drugs?
3. What other drugs is he taking?
4. What are his smoking and drinking habits?
5. Is he prone to dyspepsia? Has he had a peptic ulcer? Has he had haematemesis or malaena? Has he had a barium meal and if so why?
6. Has he ever had kidney or liver disease or a disorder of the blood?
7. What does he expect from the drug he is about to take and what has he heard about it?

WHAT TO TELL THE PATIENT

It is always wise to tell the patient something about his drug, when and how to take it and what good effects he may hope for. It is also sensible to warn him of toxic effects but not to dwell on them in too much detail because if you do so to an anxious or introspective patient the effects are almost bound to occur.

Drug interactions have been discussed earlier in this chapter. Many are reported but, happily, few produce serious results, though interactions with anticoagulant drugs may prove the exception to the rule. The NSAIDs as a class are all bound to protein (albumin) and can be displaced by more firmly protein-bound drugs or themselves displace the other drug, thus increasing or decreasing the effect of one or other or both agents.

ONE OR TWO DRUGS?

In other branches of medicine, notably in the treatment of tuberculosis or malignant disease, effective treatment demands the administration of two or more drugs at the same time in order to obtain a greater impact on the disease and to lessen the likelihood that drug resistance will develop. There is, as yet, no evidence that giving full doses of two NSAIDs has any useful additive effect. Although this question has not been fully explored, what usually seems to happen is that therapeutic effects are little changed, whereas unwanted effects increase. However, for patients who have severe night pain or early morning stiffness – as is often the case in rheumatoid arthritis and ankylosing spondylitis – it is a common practice to increase the evening dose of the NSAID or add a different agent to cover the night hours. Indomethacin 75–100 mg by mouth or suppository, taken on retiring is a popular and effective drug for this purpose.

PRACTICAL POINTS

● Most NSAIDs are effective for most rheumatic conditions provided that the patient can tolerate them in full doses.

● For short-term treatment, as in gout, full doses are needed to abort the attack in its early stages. Indomethacin, naproxen and azapropazone are all popular, but most of the NSAIDs are effective in full doses.

● For more prolonged therapy, as in rheumatoid arthritis, tolerance is as important as effectiveness; and both are more important than the convenience of only having to take the drug once or twice a day.

● Aspirin, which many consider to be the best drug for starting treatment, needs repeated administration and has other disadvantages. It can cause severe dizziness and impaired hearing with the high dosage needed for good effect; and gastro-intestinal upsets are quite common, although these can be lessened by use of an enteric-coated preparation or a different form, such as aloxiprin – a compound of aluminium oxide and aspirin.

● The best starting drug is probably naproxen, piroxicam or fenbufen, all of which are usually effective and well tolerated. If the first choice proves ineffective during a two to three week trial, a change can be made to indomethacin or any of the other drugs listed here, subject to tolerance and any history of reactions. Flurbiprofen is also effective but may cause gastro-intestinal upset, like any of the NSAIDs.

● Patients with osteoarthrosis are usually older and inflammation is a less prominent feature of their disability. Tolerance and analgesia are therefore usually more important than the anti-inflammatory properties of the drug to be chosen. Indomethacin, however, has given great help to very many patients with osteoarthrosis of the hip and knee. Naproxen, piroxicam, azapropazone or fenbufen can be tried if indomethacin is poorly tolerated. Ibuprofen is not a powerful drug but it is usually well tolerated.

● Practitioners are well advised to settle for their own lists of about six agents and gain their own experience of them. If a safe cure or even a much more effective palliative for rheumatoid arthritis is ever invented, the news of it will fly on its own wings long before any representative can bring it.

30
Corticosteroid therapy in the rheumatic diseases

Corticosteroids are the most powerful of the anti-inflammatory agents that are available for the treatment of rheumatic disease. Like the NSAIDs (see Chapter 29) they have no curative effect on the underlying pathological process but merely suppress the inflammatory features of the disease. They have no central analgesic effect but may cause euphoria or an exaggeration of the patient's mental state, either manic or depressive, particularly in high dosage.

Cortisone and hydrocortisone are less suitable for anti-inflammatory use than are their successors, which have a less potent sodium-retaining action. Prednisone and prednisolone are the corticosteroids most widely used in rheumatological practice today. Roughly equivalent oral doses are cortisone 25 mg, hydrocortisone (cortisol) 20 mg, prednisone or prednisolone 5 mg, methyl prednisolone and triamcinolone 4 mg, paramethasone 2 mg and dexamethasone and betamethasone 0.75 mg.

EFFECTS OF CORTICOSTEROIDS

Corticosteroids prevent or suppress the features of inflammation, local heat, redness, swelling and tenderness. At microscopic level they inhibit not only the features of inflammation such as capillary dilation, oedema, leucocyte migration into the inflamed area and phagocytic activity, but also such later manifestations as capillary proliferation, deposition of collagen, fibroblast proliferation and, even later, formation of scar tissue.[1] This anti-inflammatory effect is nonspecific and is exerted whatever the cause of the inflammation, whether it is mechanical, infective, allergic, chemical or immunological.

The effect of the corticosteroids on the inflammatory process is complex. There is evidence that they inhibit the release of arachidonic acid from phospholipids and thereby decrease formation of prostaglandins and related substances. They are therefore potentially dangerous if the cause of the inflammatory process is infective because they have no antibiotic action and may aggravate infections by facilitating the spread of viruses or bacteria. The steroid-treated patient is at constant risk of intercurrent infection. Corticosteroids are also potentially dangerous because they affect almost all body processes to some extent and because, at all but the smallest doses, they exert a suppressive effect on adrenocortical function with reduced response to stresses of all kinds.

The corticosteroids are powerful physiological tools which should only be used to suppress the inflammatory features of certain conditions. There is no set dose range but unwanted effects increase with higher dosage and most of the adverse effects reported are produced at levels above 10–20 mg of prednisolone daily or its equivalent (see page 199). The commoner adverse effects are listed in the Table below.

Adverse effects of systemic corticosteroid dosage

● Endocrine	Features of Cushing's syndrome: moon face, obesity, increased growth of fine hair. Suppression of growth in children. Glycosuria and hyperglycaemia. Amenorrhoea.
● Skin	Acne. Skin and subcutaneous tissue atrophy. Purpura of forearms.
● Reduced resistance to infection	
● Gastro-intestinal	Exacerbation of peptic and other ulceration. Perforation of peptic ulcer or diverticulae.
● Muscles	Myopathy.
● Eyes	Posterior subcapsular cataract. Glaucoma. Papilloedema.
● CNS	Intracranial hypertension. Mental and mood changes.
● Bone and joint	Osteoporosis. Aseptic necrosis.
● Electrolyte disturbances	Sodium and fluid retention (more with cortisol and cortisone than with later corticosteroids). Hypokalaemia.
● Withdrawal effects on reducing or stopping dosage	Signs of adrenal suppression: lethargy, hypotension, flare of suppressed disease and diminished ability to cope with stresses in all forms.

By reducing the inflammatory reaction corticosteroids reduce pain and swelling, particularly in the early morning, and improve function and the range of movement. They are therefore most useful in the treatment of the inflammatory anthropathies although they are less satisfactory than the NSAIDs in the treatment of gout. Any dosage above 6–7 mg prednisolone daily is liable to cause some degree of adrenocortical suppression and some feature of overdosage. Such a dose seldom produces dramatic improvement in rheumatoid arthritis although it is very effective in controlling polymyalgia rheumatica. There is no evidence that corticosteroids at any dosage can reverse erosive changes or prevent their occurrence.

RHEUMATIC CONDITIONS SUITABLE FOR CORTICOSTEROID THERAPY

Rheumatoid arthritis

A single systemic dose of a corticosteroid can be given in the morning or the evening and may help to reduce morning stiffness. An evening dose produces more adreno-cortical suppression than a morning dose. While no dramatic effect can be expected from 7.5 mg of prednisolone daily, whether in single or divided doses, it may give useful help in some cases if it is allied with NSAIDs and physical treatment.

In acute inflammatory episodes a higher dosage may be given, using 20–30 mg of prednisolone daily and reducing it gradually as the condition improves. However, this mode of treatment has a way of leading to prolonged high dosage with the inevitable appearance of unwanted effects. It is not uncommon practice today to give a double dose on the mornings of alternate days as this produces less adrenocortical suppression than daily dosage; but in many cases where acute inflammatory disease is present the disease tends to escape from control during the latter half of the second day if alternate dosage is used.

If corticosteroids are used with discretion they can still be a moderately useful tool in the treatment of rheumatoid arthritis, but used with indiscretion or intermittently in fluctuating doses they can have serious adverse effects. (See also Chapters 10 and 28.)

Seronegative inflammatory arthropathies

Corticosteroids may help in the ways and dosages that have been mentioned in the previous section, but they are seldom needed. They have never been popular for the treatment of ankylosing spondylitis in Great Britain. (See also Chapter 10.)

Systemic lupus erythematosus (SLE)

Corticosteroids are necessary in all but the mildest cases. They may be life-saving in acute exacerbations of the disease particularly, according to Christian[2] in lupus glomerulonephritis, in neurological involvement, in acute vasculitis, in cardio-pulmonary disease and when toxic symptoms occur with fever or when there is severe haemolytic anaemia.

In these acute and often dangerous situations a daily dose of 50–75 mg prednisolone is needed. Higher doses are often no more effective and they usually prove more toxic. Dosage can be reduced gradually as the disease comes under control. The average maintenance dose is now about 8–14 mg prednisolone, less than was considered necessary a few years ago, but dosage has to be gauged by symptomatic control in each case.

Recently so-called pulse therapy has been used in SLE. Intravenous infusions of 1 g methyl prednisolone in 500 ml of normal saline are given over four hours on three successive days.[3]

Polyarteritis nodosa

As with SLE (above) the daily dose is about 50–75 mg prednisolone in situations where life is threatened, with gradual reduction as the patient improves, although this is something that does not always happen. When corticosteroids are given later in the disease they may aggravate any hypertension that is present.

Dermatomyositis and polymyositis

The usual starting dose is around 40–60 mg prednisolone daily, although a larger dose is sometimes needed at first. Improvement is assessed by increase in muscle strength and reduction in serum enzyme levels (creatinine kinase and aldolase). Maintenance dosage is usually 5–10 mg daily. Patients with Sjögren's syndrome or an underlying neoplasm do less well, and a temporary improvement may be followed by worsening while still under treatment. (See also Chapter 20.)

Progressive systemic sclerosis (scleroderma)

Corticosteroid treatment is much less successful here but it may improve the myositic and other inflammatory features early in this disease if given in the dosage suggested for polymyositis (above), or somewhat lower.

Polymyalgia rheumatica and giant cell arteritis

Corticosteroids are the drugs of choice. Treatment of these conditions is described in Chapter 13.

LOCAL INJECTIONS OF CORTICOSTEROIDS

Injection of a corticosteroid into an inflamed joint, preferably after aspiration, will often benefit the patient as a whole, and not merely the joint treated, because the condition of that one joint is holding back his entire progress (see Chapter 31). The transient rise of corticosteroid level in the general circulation may also bring general if temporary benefit without causing any undesirable effect.

It is wise to give such injections occasionally – to break a vicious inflammatory circle – rather than regularly. The risk of infection is usually slight. Any inflamed joint in rheumatoid or seronegative arthritis is a candidate for such treatment, which is usually given to a knee, elbow or shoulder but may be used on smaller joints and wrists. Injections may also be given into painful muscular lesions such as tennis or golfer's elbow. Suitable preparations are listed in the Table on page 220. Amounts given will vary from 2 to 40 mg or even more, depending on the size of the joint and on the agent used.

Corticotrophin and tetracosactrin

Human corticotrophin (ACTH) is a peptide of thirty-nine amino-acid residues. Its main activity depends on the first twenty-four amino-acids of the peptide chain and these are the same in humans, pigs, sheep and cows. The corticotrophin that we use therapeutically is derived from the pituitaries of those animals.

Corticotrophin is inactive when taken by mouth but if it is given intramuscularly in doses up to 80 iu it stimulates the adrenal cortex to secrete more cortisol, cortico-sterone, aldosterone and some weak androgenic substances. The effect is similar to that of giving a corticosteroid by mouth and the side-effects are the same although there is a greater incidence of hypertension, acne, sodium-loading, hyperkalaemia, alkalosis and left-heart strain.

Hypersensitivity reactions may occur and prolonged use leads to the development of antibodies. When hypersensitivity reactions do occur beneficial effects lessen rapidly. Injections of ACTH are given intramuscularly once daily and usually in doses of 10–40 iu.

Tetracosactrin is a synthetic analogue of corticotrophin. It contains the first twenty-four of the thirty-nine amino-acids and has the same therapeutic activity, 1 mg of tetracosactrin having roughly the same clinical effect as 100–150 iu of corticotrophin. A total dose higher than 1 mg a week intramuscularly, whether given daily or at intervals of a few days, will produce Cushingoid overdosage effects if it is continued for more than a few weeks and I prefer to give 0.1 or 0.15 mg daily.

Injections of corticotrophin or tetracosactrin are given in courses of ten to fourteen days or more to control acute inflammatory episodes in a polyarthritis that does not respond to other measures. Such treatment may be rarely needed to control an attack of acute gout that has persisted in spite of full NSAID therapy. Antibodies may develop and local reactions occur in some cases.

STOPPING TREATMENT

Corticosteroids should never be stopped suddenly or tapered off very rapidly. Reduction must always be gradual and slow in order to avoid the 'withdrawal syndrome', a mixture of features of adrenocortical suppression and exacerbation of symptoms of the suppressed disease.

PRACTICAL POINTS

- Corticosteroids are the most potent anti-inflammatory drugs used to treat the rheumatic diseases. They may be helpful in:
  - —SLE
  - —Polyarteritis nodosa
  - —Dermatomyositis and polymyositis
  - —Scleroderma
  - —Polymyalgia rheumatica
  - —Giant cell arteritis
  - —Rheumatoid arthritis
  - —Seronegative arthropathies (rarely).
- Corticosteroids should never be used if the cause of the inflammatory process is infective.
- Corticosteroids may reduce patients' responses to stress by causing adrenocortical suppression.
- The occasional injection of a corticosteroid into an inflamed joint may help to break the vicious inflammatory circle and so benefit the patient as a whole.
- Reduction of corticosteroid therapy must always be gradual. It must never be stopped abruptly.

31

Aspiration and injection for diagnosis and treatment

ASPIRATION

If there is any doubt about the diagnosis, a joint may be aspirated to obtain fluid for microscopy and culture. Aspiration is essential if pyarthrosis is suspected (see Chapter 5) and is useful when there is a possibility of gout or pseudogout in a large joint (see Chapter 12). If a joint has become rapidly distended within an hour or less, haemorrhage is probably the cause. Distension that develops over a period of two to twenty-four hours suggests an acute synovial reaction to injury or the deposition of crystals. More insidious distension is usually due to a low-grade reaction to infection or trauma, or to a noninfective inflammatory arthropathy such as rheumatoid arthritis. The Table below gives the usual findings in different conditions.

Synovial fluid aspirates

	Normal	Noninflammatory or traumatic	RA and sterile inflammatory	Septic arthritis	Acute crystal arthropathy
Appearance	Clear	Clear	Often turbid	Turbid	Clear with fibrin features
Colour	White or yellow	Yellow	Yellow/green	Brown/green	Yellow
Viscosity	High	High	Low	Low	Low
Clots			●	●	●
Approx white blood cells (× 10)	<200	500–1,000	30,000 (2,000–75,000)	100,000 (60,000+)	20,000–60,000
Crystals					●
Culture				●	
Predominant cell	Mononuclears	Mononuclears	Neutrophils	Neutrophils	Neutrophils

ASPIRATION AND JOINT INJECTION

The best sites for aspiration of a joint or for injection of an antibiotic into it are:

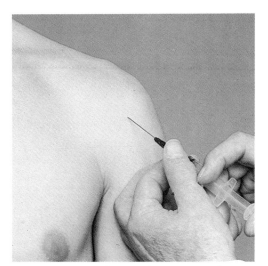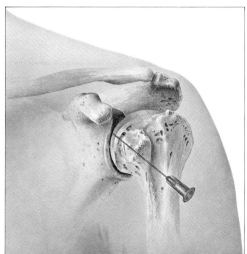

Figure 80 a, b; (*Below* 81a, b)   **Shoulder (patient sitting)**

1. Glenohumeral – just below and lateral to the coracoid process from in front or, preferably, from behind.

2. Acromioclavicular – anterolateral approach.

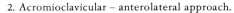

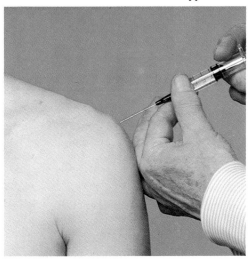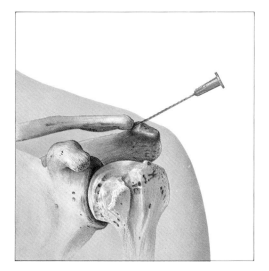

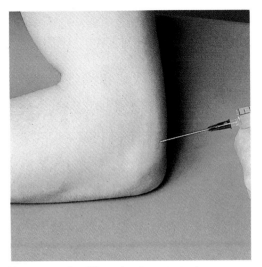
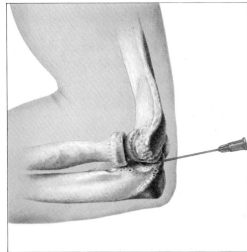

Figure 82a, b Elbow (patient sitting)

With elbow flexed to 90°, 1 cm above and 1 cm behind the lateral condyle. The needle is directed medially and slightly downwards.

Figure 83a, b Wrist (patient sitting)

With palm downwards. Inject downwards, just below ulnar styloid.

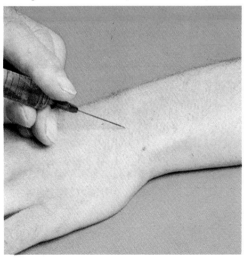
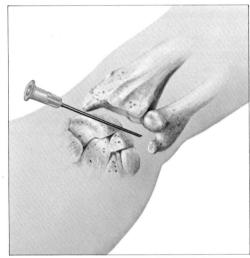

Complications

It is unusual for aspiration or injection to be complicated by haemorrhage or sepsis. Tissues may be damaged by repeated injections of corticosteroid or of large amounts of fluid into a small joint. Injection of crystalline corticosteroid may produce a pseudogout reaction. The joint should be rested for twelve to twenty-four hours after aspiration or injection of a corticosteroid or antibiotic. The patient must be told to report any painful or inflammatory reaction that lasts for more than a few hours.

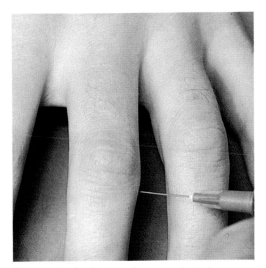 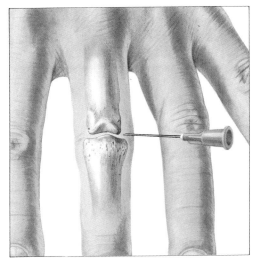

Figure 84a, b   Fingers (patient sitting)

Medial or lateral side of dorsal surface of MPs or PIPs.

Figure 85a, b   Hip (patient lying)

2 cm below inguinal ligament, just lateral to femoral artery. Inject downwards and slightly medially.

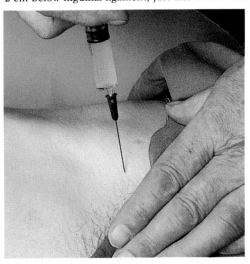 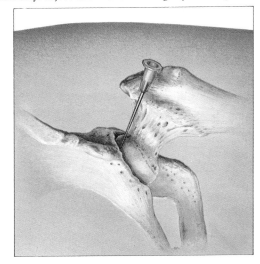

Corticosteroids

Corticosteroid injections are given to break a vicious inflammatory circle and should not, as a rule, be repeated into any one joint more than three times within a period of six months. They may also be given to assist the moblization of a painful 'stuck' joint. A useful mixture is equal parts of 1 per cent lignocaine and a corticosteroid solution (see Table overleaf). The amount of fluid to be injected varies between 0.25–0.5 ml for an acromioclavicular or finger joint and 10 ml for a glenohumeral joint.

Corticosteroids for local intra-articular and soft-tissue injections

—hydrocortisone (as acetate) 25 mg per ml
—prednisolone (as acetate) 25 mg per ml
—prednisolone (as tertiary butyl acetate)
  20 mg per ml
—prednisolone (as pivalate) 50 mg per ml
—prednisolone (as sodium phosphate)
  16 mg per ml

—methylprednisolone (as acetate)
  40 mg per ml
—triamcinolone (as acetate)
  10 and 40 mg per ml
—triamcinolone (as hexacetonide)
  20 mg per ml
—dexamethasone (as sodium phosphate)
  4 or 5 mg per ml

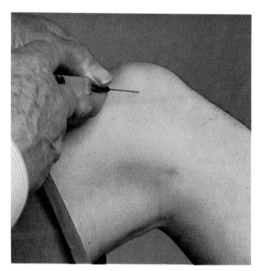
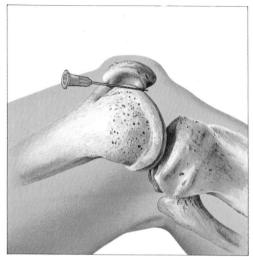

Figure 86a, b   Knee (patient lying)
Knee slightly flexed. On medial side below patella, with needle pointing downwards and slightly laterally.

Figure 87a, b   Ankle (patient lying)
Anteromedial to anterior malleolus, needle pointing downwards and slightly laterally.

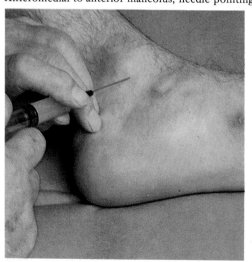
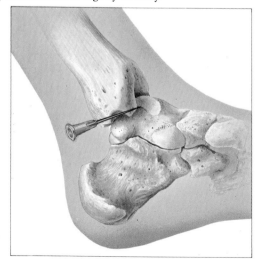

EXTRA-ARTICULAR INJECTIONS

Injections may also be given into painful extra-articular tissues.

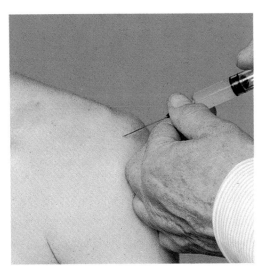 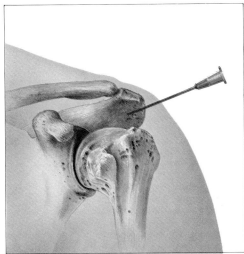

Figure 88a, b   Subacromial bursae

Inject from the side between acromium and head of humerus, aiming towards the head of the humerus. Use 5 ml of 1 per cent lignocaine and 20–40 mg of hydrocortisone acetate or triamcinolone hexacetonide.

Figure 89a, b   Carpal tunnel compression (the median nerve is coloured red in this diagram).

Inject in crease of wrist on palmar aspect, just lateral to the midline, pointing the needle inwards and slightly towards the palm. Use a fine-bore needle, do not go more than 5–9 mm below the skin, and do not inject more than 1 ml of lignocaine-corticosteroid mixture. Note that the median nerve lies under the palmaris longus if present (the muscle is absent in some people). Numbness of the thumb and adjacent finger suggests you have hit the nerve.

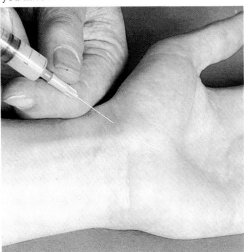 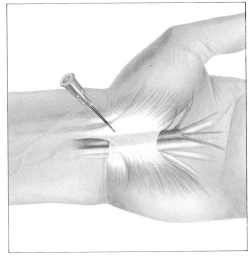

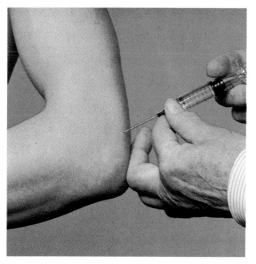 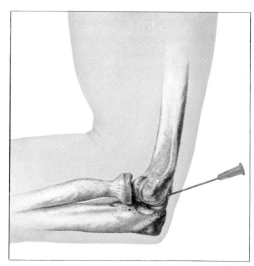

Figure 90a, b   Tennis elbow (lateral epicondylitis)

Inject 2–3 ml of lignocaine-corticosteroid mixture into the muscle origin at the tender spot. Inject on to bone. This injection is often very painful.

Figure 91a, b   Golfer's elbow (medial epicondylitis)

Inject as above but into the flexor origin at the medial humeral epicondyle.

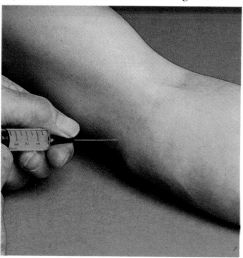 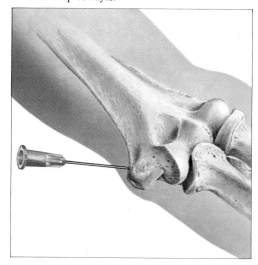

Tender spots (pain points)

These may be injected with local anaesthetic or a mixture of corticosteroid solution and local anaesthetic.

Complications

Grateful patients are not always the rule. Injections often break pain cycles but not always, and the effect is temporary in most cases. Infections and haemorrhages do

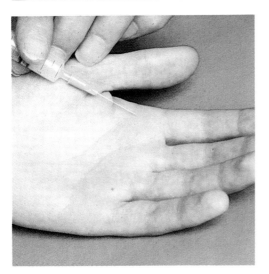
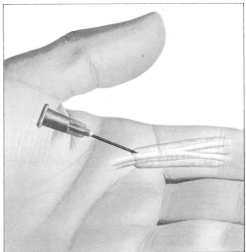

Figure 92a, b   Trigger finger
Injecting flexor tendon of index finger.

Figure 93a, b
Injecting abductor pollicis longus at wrist. Inject not into tendon but into sheath alongside, below the extensor retinaculum.

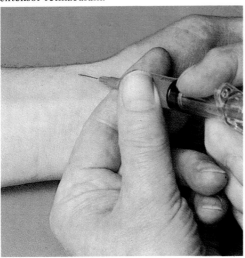
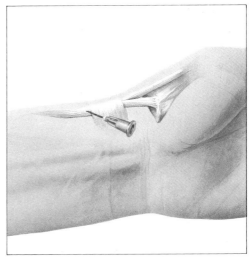

occur, even if they are rare. Pain may be exacerbated for a time, sometimes severely, as with some epicondylar injections, and sometimes for long periods if nervous tissue has been injected.

Misplaced injections may damage tissues and injections into muscles and ligaments may cause them to rupture even if the tendon is a large one like the tendon of Achilles. Overuse of a limb after an injection has eased the pain may do more harm than good in the long run.

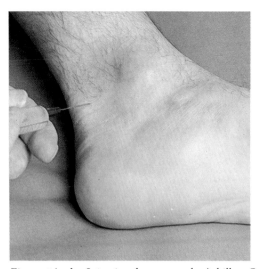 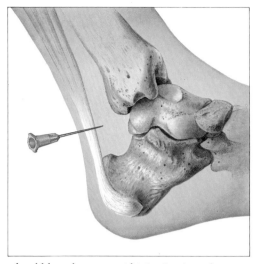

Figure 94a, b   Injecting deep to tendo Achilles. Care should be taken to avoid injecting into the tendon itself.

Figure 95a, b   Injecting suprasinatus tendinitis.

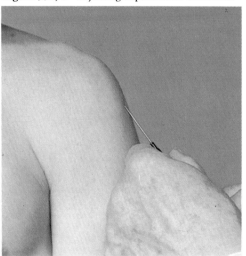 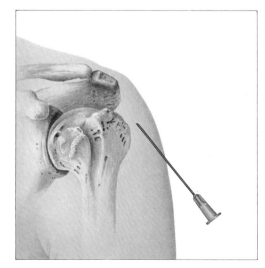

LOCAL TENDINITIS

The muscle tendons and their sheaths may be affected by the disease process in rheumatoid and some other forms of arthritis, as well as in some other disorders including tuberculosis. Many forms of tendinitis, however, are localized to one area outside the joint capsule and are not part of any systemic disease. In such cases local therapy may be a great help.

Trigger finger

Trigger finger is due to tenosynovitis of the flexor tendons of the fingers, with a nodular expansion of the tendon catching in its sheath. It may only affect one finger, which locks in flexion and gives a click when forcibly straightened by the other hand. This condition may be associated with trauma, often repetitive, but there is usually no obvious cause. Trigger finger may correct itself with the help of local rubs such as old-fashioned iodine ointment, hot hand soaks and exercises. It may need an injection of hydrocortisone into the sheath (but not into the tendon which may rupture if injected). A minor operation for surgical release is sometimes necessary.

Trigger thumb

This is a condition similar to trigger finger, affecting the tendon of flexor pollicis longus.

De Quervain's tenosynovitis

This affects the abductor pollicis longus or extensor pollicis brevis tendons at the wrist. It is a common condition often related to repeated trauma, particular in women. Use of the thumb is painful and tenderness is usually maximal in the 'anatomical snuff-box' between and over these tendons. Forced ulnar deviation with the thumb grasped in the palm by the patient's fingers causes pain at the lesion in the tendon sheath. If the thumb is abducted against resistance the tendons stand out and the painful spot can be located.

Fill a 2 ml syringe with 1 per cent lignocaine and use a no. 20 needle. Insert the needle obliquely along the line of the tendon at a point just distal to the tender spot. With a finger on the tendon proximal to the skin puncture advance the needle and inject lignocaine slowly to blow up the sheath. Leave the needle in place and inject 1 ml (25 mg) of hydrocortisone solution into the sheath. This is not a painful procedure and is usually successful.

Achilles tendinitis

This condition must be distinguished from an acute injury of the tendon which should be treated by rest or, if rupture is complete, by surgery. Otherwise conservative measures are usually sufficient. The heel of the shoe may be raised by a cobbler or a calcaneal pad may be inserted. Resistant cases may be associated with subtendinous bursitis. A corticosteroid solution can be infiltrated around the tender area but never into the tendon itself.

Supraspinatus tendinitis

This is a common lesion of the shoulder, most often found in middle-aged men. The condition may be precipitated by mild trauma or exertion, although there is often a past history of recurrent shoulder pain. The pain may be worse at night and interfere with sleep. A painful arc from 70 to 100° on abduction is characteristic (see page 16).

This often responds to injection. The patient sits with the affected arm hanging down loosely. Palpate the gap between the humeral head and the acromion. Mark the spot. Inject 2 ml of 1 per cent lignocaine at a depth of about 2.5 cm. Withdraw the needle to allow the local anaesthetic to act. When it has done so the shoulder can be moved freely without pain. Now inject 2 ml of corticosteroid solution into the same area. There may be pain for some hours after the injection. This treatment may have to be repeated after a few days.

Bicipital tendinitis or tenosynovitis

Tenderness is maximal in the bicipital groove of the head of the humerus. Rotate the arm externally and mark the skin over the area of maximal tenderness. Inject 2 ml of 1 per cent lignocaine along the groove but not into the tendon. Resistance will be slight so long as the needle remains in the synovial sheath. Do not remove the needle but use it to inject 2 ml of corticosteroid solution. There may be after-pain but it is less severe than that which follows supraspinatus tendon injection (see above) and seldom lasts as long.

Prognosis

Tendinitis is sometimes occupational and sometimes due to trauma which is often minor and repeated, but there may be no apparent cause. It can be very painful and interfere with work and pleasure, but usually gets better quite soon if it is not part of a systemic disease such as rheumatoid arthritis. The fact that it may be the first manifestation of such a disease makes a cautious prognosis advisable. Most cases settle in time if treated either conservatively with no injections, or with a single injection, or two injections at most in the same area. More frequent injection is less likely to help and more likely to damage the tendon.

32
Rest and exercise

Rest and exercise are powerful therapeutic weapons that should be used with care and tailored individually. They can produce great benefits, but they also have drawbacks and risks, like all other powerful therapeutic measures.

ABSOLUTE REST

One of the most difficult decisions that have to be made during the management of arthritic and rheumatic conditions is when to rest the patient absolutely, when to rest him partially under set rules, when to allow him to move freely and when to encourage him to be active beyond his inclination.

The label ABSOLUTE REST used to hang over the beds of sanitorium patients with tuberculosis in those prewar days when rest in a sanitorium with full nutrition was the only treatment available for this disease and the curative powers of rest were strongly emphasized in such famous books as Hilton's *Rest and Pain*.

I remember a tuberculous patient at a London hospital in the 1930s who asked his eminent physician what treatment he was going to have, only to be told, both briefly and forcibly, that he was already having the best treatment possible which was absolute rest. Just lying still in bed was Treatment with a capital T, although those with pulmonary infection might have a pneumothorax or a thoracoplasty to enforce additional local rest, and those with disease of the spine or a long bone were encased in plaster of Paris.

There were, in those days, many resemblances between the tuberculous and the arthritic disorders. Both were chronic, crippling, inflammatory diseases with no specific curative treatment, although one was potentially lethal and the other was not. Both caused much ill-health and inability to work. They were so similar in some of their clinical and histological features that the same treatments were often used, including analgesics, antipyretics, injections of gold salts and, above all, rest. Many arthritic patients underwent long periods of rest; some were improved by it, others were not.

REST: PROS AND CONS

Before considering the value of rest in the modern management of arthritis, it is helpful to look at its pros and cons.

Bed rest for arthritis

Pros	Cons
● Reduction of swelling	● Risk of thrombophlebitis and embolism
● Reduction of pain	● Increased osteoporosis
● Maintenance of correct position	● Risk of bedsores
● Reduction in repeated small traumata	● Increased stiffening
● Gain in weight	● Muscle wasting
● Possible resolution of inflammatory process	● Renal stones
	● Deterioration of morale
● Improvement of morale	● Depression.

A programme of graded rest/activity has to be decided upon for every individual and will depend on the patient's general condition, his local articular condition and his mental attitude. The physician, orthopaedic surgeon, nurses and therapists will all have their views about how much or how little he should do, and the patient, who usually has his own view and often knows better than anyone, will steer his way through these islands of independent opinion.

In the field of rheumatology we are not, as a rule, dealing with a potentially lethal malady and must remember that the importance of maintaining function is as great as that of reducing inflammation. If a patient with ankylosing spondylitis is treated as though he had spinal tuberculosis with no antibiotics available, he will probably suffer less pain but will certainly end up being much less mobile and may well be completely ankylosed in spine, neck and hip.

The following are general guides to the use of rest in the management of certain arthritic disorders. They must not, however, be applied as rules of thumb in every case. Each patient in each disease group presents an individual psychophysical problem.

OSTEOARTHROSIS

The aim is to preserve the fullest possible mobility although it may be frustrated by the poor cardiac or pulmonary function of some patients. Any exacerbation of symptoms after exercise in the affected weight-bearing joint or joints is acceptable if it lasts for an hour or so, but if it lasts for two hours or more too much has been attempted, and if it lasts until the following day much too much was attempted. Effusion in a knee can be evidence of overuse.

On the other hand, increased pain and stiffness in weight-bearing joints may set in after only thirty to ninety minutes of immobility in the same position, and all affected joints should be put through their full range of movements every hour at least. Distances walked should be as long as pain permits, subject to the one-hour rule. Drugs taken to relieve pain will often increase the range and there is seldom any subsequent sign of overuse in the affected joint. Our analgesics and NSAIDs are not so efficient as to produce a real Charcot's joint (see page 43).

Osteoarthrotic patients who are highly motivated and have a low pain threshold seem to do better than others. A desire to do something and a pleasure in doing it appear to have pain-relieving properties of their own. Nevertheless, acute painful episodes may call for periods of partial or complete rest. Aspiration of the joint and possibly injection of a corticosteroid may shorten the period of incapacity during which weight-bearing has to be reduced or abandoned. Acute painful episodes in the cervical or lumbar spine may necessitate complete rest, with analgesics and sometimes with sedatives as well.

Although osteoarthrosis is pathologically a chronic and irreversible condition, the symptoms are not. Even in the worst-seeming joints symptoms may change and lessen. Quite often the bad hip becomes the good hip and vice versa. The factors that produce the pain are variable and do not necessarily parallel the pathological progress of the disease. There must therefore be a flexible attitude to the use of rest and immobility, with the fullest activity that is possible in terms of pain tolerance and stricter rest only in acute painful, traumatic or inflammatory episodes.

The time for surgery on hip or knee is the time when pain and loss of function have made life intolerable. If the patient knows what surgery has to offer and its possible complications, he can tell you when this time has come. Some practitioners in countries with State-run health services try to foresee this stage and make an earlier reference, knowing that patients are likely to wait many months for consultation and very many more for operation.

RHEUMATOID ARTHRITIS

Most rheumatoid patients will improve with rest and without change of drugs. Active disease is often sustained in a rheumatoid joint by a degree of physical activity that is only slightly greater than its capacity and I have repeatedly seen patients' active disease settle down when they are given time off work or put to rest in bed, their joints becoming less swollen, less painful and more mobile.

When the disease is first diagnosed, it is probably best – unless it is mild or is affecting only a few joints – to admit the patient to hospital for two to three weeks in order to educate him in his own therapy. He should begin with bed rest, appropriate exercises and drugs, resting the active joints in splints which can be removed for periods of gentle exercises. Then he should be gradually mobilized with physiotherapy and more exercises. When he goes home he should have a period of convalescence before returning to work which should be modified at first. A shorter working day, say from 10 am to 4 pm, will tax him less and save him from the rigours of rush-hour travel. A full working day may become possible later.

Many rheumatoid sufferers are busy house-wives. When they are returning home from hospital they should be advised to rest for half to one hour in midmorning, and one to two hours during the afternoon. This will help to guard them against the rapid return of symptoms that so often afflicts the house-proud. As time passes, domestic duties may be increased and rest periods shortened. Only the patient herself truly knows what is too much for her in the way of activity. Although measurable improvement does occur in joints that are adequately rested and although deterioration occurs in those that are overworked, a mind occupied with congenial duties is less aware of pain. So it is that many patients prefer to work even when they are exhausted by 4 pm and every joint is aching badly.

There have been attempts to compare the value of hospital rest with modified-rest and no-rest regimes but results have been rather inconclusive. As a general rule it can be said that bed rest with splintage and a programme of exercises is useful in very active cases, that modification of activity will suffice in less active disease and that those whose malady is relatively inactive need do no more than avoid extreme exertion.

Life is for living and rheumatoid arthritis is often an unremitting chronic condition, so compromises must be made. While rest relieves pain, boredom often aggravates it. Rest or no rest, it is important to keep the mind active. Any work, hobby or social activity that seems worth while to the patient deserves to be encouraged so long as it does not involve a greater physical strain than she and her arthritis can tolerate.

ANKYLOSING SPONDYLITIS

In the 1920s and 1930s and particularly in places where this was thought to be a rheumatoid disorder, ankylosing spondylitis was treated by rest and plaster jackets or braces, in the belief that the inflammation would settle down leaving the patient with a straight spine instead of a fixed kyphosis. A good position was indeed achieved in some cases but only at the expense of mobility. Spine, hips, neck and sometimes shoulders all became ankylosed, rigid and functionally ineffective.

Orthodox therapy between the two wars was based on orthopaedic notions of immobilization and posture rather than on exercise, pain relief and preservation of function. This was disastrous. The patients who did best were those who kept active, took analgesics and stayed away from orthopaedic surgeons. The bad treatment resulted from overconfidence in rest as a form of therapy and the unfortunate transatlantic and nonEuropean idea that this disorder was a variant of rheumatoid arthritis. If a disease has a different pathology and a different prognosis, with a greater incidence in a different sex and a different age group, it would seem more logical to observe and listen to the sufferer than to classify him on the biopsy histological evidence of a peripheral joint in a disorder primarily affecting the spine. The essential feature of this disease is its tendency to cause ankylosis and this tendency is enhanced by rest.

Mobility, not rest, is the key to the treatment of ankylosing spondylitis, which cripples by arthrodesis. The patient must have adequate medication to suppress the pain that restricts mobility and he must be kept moving. This rule applies to spine, hips, shoulders, neck and thorax, all of which tend to fuse if they are immobile. The peripheral joints may be damaged by overuse but they are usually only affected transiently and are, in any case, less important than the spinal articulations in this disease.

The only exceptions to this rule are those who:

1. are undergoing a very acute painful crisis (these are uncommon),
2. have suffered acute trauma, or
3. have an area of painful mobility between two fused segments of the spine.

The same principles apply in the ankylosing spondylopathies of psoriasis, enteropathic arthritis and Reiter's disease. In these disorders the peripheral joints may be more seriously affected than the spinal joints, particularly at an early stage of the disease. If and when spondylitis appears, the first aim of treatment must be to arrest the ankylosing process in spine and girdle joints.

THE SERONEGATIVE ARTHROPATHIES

Other than various ankylosing spondylarthropathies, these need a modified rest programme depending on symptoms and assisted by analgesics and NSAIDs.

Colitic or Crohn's arthropathy

Peripheral joints are affected less chronically and less persistently than they are in rheumatoid arthritis (see page 22) and apart from acute inflammatory episodes, rest need only be related to the joint symptoms present at the time. Symptoms tend to wax and wane, sometimes exacerbating with those of colitis.

Reiter's disease

Initial symptoms (see Chapter 5) may be very severe, particularly in knees, ankles and feet. They may be very much worse than in the average case of rheumatoid arthritis and sometimes almost as severe as in gout. Rest is essential because weight-bearing is too painful to allow anything else, but in most cases this acute phase settles in a few weeks and mobilization can begin, the need for rest being dictated solely by the severity of the symptoms.

In about a third of cases symptoms abate within a few weeks or months and never return. In another third they remit and exacerbate for several months, while in the remainder they become chronic in some joints only. About 20 per cent develop the picture of ankylosing spondylitis. The need to advise rest varies widely from one case to another. The aim is to control swelling and discomfort by local and systemic treatment. Splintage is seldom necessary.

Psoriatic arthropathy

The same rules apply as for Reiter's disease (above). This condition is usually milder and less diffuse than rheumatoid arthritis. Its severity does not run parallel with that of the skin disease. A condition that resembles ankylosing spondylitis occurs in about 10 per cent, with an equal sex distribution. Some rare unfortunates are affected in both spinal and peripheral joints and the attitude to rest must be an empirical compromise because spinal stiffness calls for maximum mobility but painful weight-bearing joints may make it impossible.

GOUT

Chronic tophaceous gout is receding into history. The patient with acute gout will make his own decisions about rest, refusing to put foot to ground so long as the attack lasts but walking to the office or golf course as soon as it is over.

SYSTEMIC LUPUS ERYTHEMATOSUS

SLE is a chronic disease whose management depends on the severity of the systemic process rather than on the local joint changes. When it is very acute bed rest is essential. When it is subacute, activity must be modified. When it is fully controlled the patient can lead a controlled life with only modest restriction of overpositive activity. In motoring terms, his can be a life in any gear except overdrive.

It must be borne in mind, however, that beneath the steroid-controlled surface of most SLE patients there is a brittle reactivity, so that infections, physical stresses, frustrations, rebuffs and even such small disturbances as a prophylactic injection may be poorly tolerated and met with aggression or despair, which may, in turn, lead to serious exacerbation of the original disease. It is a fair general rule in the management of SLE that activity is best maintained at a slightly lower level than that which would seem to be justified by the physical signs. Local joint changes are usually but not always of minor importance compared with systemic ones.

PRACTICAL POINTS

● In **osteoarthrosis** acute painful episodes can occur, and at such times rest provides relief.
● In **rheumatoid arthritis** rest has important therapeutic roles, not only during acute attacks, but in order to main good health and prevent deterioration.
● In **ankylosing spondylitis** absolute rest does more harm than good and can lead to permanent stiffness of the affected spine.
● In **Reiter's disease, SLE** and other similar conditions the degrees of pain in the joints influence the extent of rest and exercise that are possible.

33
Diet in the rheumatic diseases

When it comes to question time at the end of a lecture on rheumatic disorders to a lay audience in any part of the world it is safe to bet that one or more of the first five questions will be about diet. It is widely believed that there must be a diet for every sort of arthritis and that 'acids' and constipation must be bad for them all.

But as others[1] have already said, a huge amount of scientific investigation has failed to show that any form of nutritional deficiency or excess plays a major part in causing any form of arthritis. Walter Bauer[2] evaluated the evidence in favour of using seven different diets: no acid fruits or vegetables, only carbohydrate, protein or fat at any particular meal, alteration of acid-base ratio, omission of foods to which the patient was thought to be sensitive, low-calorie diet, low-protein diet and low-carbohydrate diet. He came to the conclusion that there was no evidence which could justify the use of any of these diets in rheumatoid arthritis. Bayles et al[3] made a careful analysis of the dietary history of thirty-one patients during the year before their first manifestations of disease and found that their nutritional intake did not differ from that of nonrheumatoid controls.

Although the evidence shows that there is almost certainly no ideal arthritic diet, there are always several popular diets going the rounds with many devoted patients who swear by them, but in the wise words of *Diet in Arthritis*,[4] published by the American Arthritis Foundation, 'Contrary to popular opinion and misinformation issued by self-appointed "experts" there is no such thing as a special arthritis diet.' There may be, however, a special Mrs Blenkinsop (who happens to have rheumatoid arthritis) diet as she is allergic to several foodstuffs, or a special Mrs Alpenstock (who happens to have psoriatic arthritis) diet as she has a very active colon, triggered into action by certain foodstuffs.

SOME UNUSUAL ARTHRITIC RESPONSES TO DIET

'Cheese arthritis'

Parke and Hughes[5] quote the case of a thirty-eight-year-old woman who was exceedingly fond of cheese and had consumed up to 450 g of it daily since her twenties.

Although she had multiple allergies and was sensitive to penicillin there was no clear history of adverse reaction to cheese. Her mother, who had rheumatoid arthritis, also reacted to penicillin, Elastoplast, detergents, aspirin and nickel, while her sister and niece both had asthma.

At the age of twenty-seven this woman developed rheumatoid arthritis. Both gold and penicillamine had to be stopped because of mucocutaneous reactions and she suffered severe gastro-intestinal discomfort on aspirin, indomethacin and azothioprine, and – like her mother – rashes related to Elastoplast and detergents. There was progressive and erosive seronegative polyarthritis, not fully controlled by prednisolone 10 mg daily. She had dryness of the eyes and mouth and a positive Schirmer's test.

This patient agreed to stop taking milk, cheese and butter but continued to eat meat. Three weeks later she began to improve. Both synovitis and morning stiffness diminished. Improvement continued with occasional relapses that occurred within twelve hours of her taking dairy products by mistake. Whenever she was 'rechallenged' with milk or Cheddar cheese, both clinical and laboratory tests showed a worsening and she developed IgE antibodies. All this happened to a person who never complained of food intolerance or manifested food allergy and whose skin tests were negative for milk antigen and only positive for cheese.

The 'Dong diet'

One of the oldest treatments for rheumatoid arthritis is starvation. Some patients improve on it but relapse when they start even a restricted diet. Such cases are exceptional. Most rheumatoid sufferers are ill-nourished and need a full rather than a restricted diet. The famous 'Dong diet' was no doubt extremely successful in Dr Dong's own case where it had the advantage of being based on Dr Dong's own multiple allergies. And it does appear to benefit some patients who may well have similar food allergies.

WHAT TO ADVISE?

Very often the benefit obtained from a special diet in any chronic arthritic disorder appears to be more in the patient taking a keen interest in getting positively involved in his own therapy than on its (often rather odd) contents. There is evidently room for further research on the dietetic side of rheumatology but little reason in the meantime to advise patients to spend money on fancy diets that have no scientific basis, however beguilingly they may be promoted in the lay press and illustrated magazines.

Some generalizations, however, can be made about diet in arthritis.

OBESITY

Patients with osteoarthrosis are often too fat. Obese osteoarthritics who cannot move about normally tend to gain weight if they do not restrict their calories. The fatter they get the more immobile they become and a vicious circle is set up. They are particularly difficult to rehabilitate after surgery or any stay in hospital.

There must be rigid restriction of fat and carbohydrate. The patient should weigh himself twice a week and record his weight on a wall chart, preferably one drawn on a large scale so that losses and gains look more impressive. He should aim at losing about 1 kg each week.

Obesity is less common in rheumatoid or seronegative polyarthritis. The sufferer from one of these diseases has often lost weight and needs to increase his calories rather than decrease them. Where obesity does complicate inflammatory polyarthritis in a patient whose activity is limited by his disease he should be advised to attempt reduction with a low-calorie diet but it must have an adequate protein, vitamin, mineral and electrolyte content.

GOUT

A similar programme of gradual weight reduction is necessary for the obese gouty patient who may precipitate an acute attack if he loses weight swiftly by means of a crash diet. The gouty subject should also restrict his intake of foods that are rich in nucleoproteins including:

- Liver
- Kidney
- Heart
- Sweetbread
- Fish roes
- Herring
- Mussels
- Sardines
- Meat extract
- Yeast
- Anchovies
- Bacon
- Codfish
- Goose
- Grouse
- Veal
- Venison
- Pheasant
- Partridge
- Pigeon

While such restrictions have only a modest effect on the blood level of uric acid, an excessive intake of one or more of them may elevate that level and precipitate an acute attack, especially if the food is washed down with strong beer, champagne or port.

Inebriety alone can precipitate an attack of gout and many patients know which drink is most likely to upset them. It is, of course, usually the one that they like best. When I lived in a mews house in London loud bangs on the left-hand party wall told me that my neighbour, a chauffeur, had taken at least three strong beers, while similar noises from the right told me that my other neighbour, a retired Royal Navy Commander, had been drinking port.

In many gouty patients attacks seem to be brought on by a break in routine. One may be made ill by too much food and drink; another by a period of fasting when there is not only reduced renal clearance of uric acid due to starvation ketosis with increase in serum β-hydroxybutyrate concentration but also an excess production of uric acid from catabolism of body protein.

WEIGHT LOSS

Loss of weight may be seen in any inflammatory polyarthritis, particularly during periods of active disease with fever and general malaise. Diarrhoea may complicate the picture and contribute to the emaciation in the arthropathies associated with Crohn's disease and ulcerative colitis. Here the diet must be adequate in calories and contain sufficient protein to offset the loss by the bowel and it must also be palatable enough to appeal to someone who is ill, anorexic and perhaps nauseated.

Although high-residue diets are now generally recommended for certain diseases of the intestines such as diverticulitis it is reasonable to limit the amount of roughage during periods of marked colonic overactivity or bleeding. A few of these patients are intolerant of dairy products, milk in particular.

SUPPLEMENTS

If steroids have been used in treatment, particularly at high dosage over long periods of time, osteoporosis is to be expected and calcium supplements may be given. Vitamin supplements may be needed in any of the inflammatory polyarthropathies, but especially in those associated with diarrhoea.

GLUTEN ENTEROPATHY AND OTHER GASTRO-INTESTINAL ARTHROPATHIES

Arthritis may occur with gluten-sensitive enteropathy (adult coeliac disease), in which the malabsorption syndrome is due to intolerance of gluten. These patients cannot tolerate cereals such as wheat, rye, oats and barley, which have a high gluten content. A gluten-free diet usually leads to improvement of the rheumatic as well as the gut manifestations but the improvement may be delayed. Supplements of vitamins D, B and K, folic acid, calcium and iron may be needed after exacerbations of the diarrhoea.

Contrary to what is firmly believed in by many older members of the lay public there is no evidence that constipation causes or even aggravates any form of arthritis, but the opposite is often true.

The arthritis that sometimes follows an intestinal by-pass operation for gross obesity and that induces chronic diarrhoea cannot be improved by diet. If antirheumatic drug treatment is ineffective it may be necessary to restore the normal anatomy of the bowel.

Patients with such connective-tissue disorders as progressive systemic sclerosis (scleroderma) and systemic lupus erythematosus (SLE) may lose weight, whether or not they have diarrhoea, but in the absence of known sensitivities these people need the same sort of diet as rheumatoids – one adequate in protein, calories and vitamins.

In the absence of a gastric or duodenal ulcer, patients with enteropathic arthropathies tolerate the usual antiarthritic drugs quite well.

FACTORS AFFECTING APPETITE AND NUTRITION

It is always necessary to remember that drugs given to arthritics may have a bad effect on nutrition. Most arthritic patients are on drugs and all NSAIDs may cause a greater or smaller degree of anorexia and/or indigestion. Some, particularly mefanamic and flufenamic acid, may cause diarrhoea. There are, on the other hand, some drugs that are given for indigestion which seem to cause arthritis or arthralgia. Recent reports accuse cimetidine, and overuse of purgatives may cause cramps and muscle aches due to deficiency of magnesium, potassium or sodium.[6]

The most likely cause of interference with nutrition, however, is the disease itself. There is dysphagia in progressive systemic sclerosis and diarrhoea in ulcerative colitis. The osteoarthrotic finds preparing food burdensome, even if someone else has done his shopping, and the rheumatoid arthritic is often ill and anorexic, quite apart from his pain and deformity.

PRACTICAL POINTS

- No nutritional deficiency or excess has been shown to play a major part in causing any common form of arthritis.
- Involving patients in the planning of their diet can itself bring beneficial effects.
- Media-promoted 'fad' diets should not be recommended.
- Obese osteoarthritics should be advised to lose weight.
- Gouty patients should be advised to restrict intake of food rich in nucleoproteins, and not to drink alcohol to excess.
- Prescribe calcium supplements for osteoporosis.
- A gluten-free diet usually helps gluten enteroarthropathy.
- NSAIDs may cause indigestion and anorexia.

Epilogue

To conclude this book I would like to suggest six golden rules for rheumatic practice: three diagnostic and three therapeutic.

1. In the face of such a wide variety of arthritic and rheumatic disorders it is essential for the physician to get the diagnosis right. He should not be content with just a main diagnosis, because other treatable disorders, from a local ligamentous tear to an anxiety or depressive state, may exist or supervene in addition to the main diagnosis.
2. A full and carefully taken history is usually of equal importance to a thorough physical examination.
3. Radiological and pathological investigations are often essential but their excessive multiplication may mislead the doctor in addition to increasing the patient's anxiety. Keep them to a minimum.
4. Bring the patient into the picture as soon as you have made your diagnosis and decided on your plan for treatment. He should be made aware of the natural history of his disease and be given detailed instructions about rest, exercise, exercises and diet. He should know how and when to take his medicines and what benefits he may hope to gain from each of them. Possible unwanted effects must be mentioned but not given too much emphasis.
5. Ensure that the patient has an active rather than a passive attitude to his treatment. It is his treatment for him to put into practice under instruction.
6. Finally, and most important of all, encourage the patient to maintain maximum mobility compatible with his arthritic condition and to keep an interest in things outside himself and his illness. The best analgesic is an occupied mind.

Notes

Chapter 2

1. KOZIN, F. in *Arthritis and Allied Conditions*, ed. McCarty, D.J. (Lea and Febiger, Philadelphia, 9th edn, 1979), 1103.
2. ROY, S., OLDHAM, R. and NICHOL, F.E., *Brit. Med. J. 284* (1982), 117.
3. STEINBROCKER, O., SPITZEN, N. and FRIEDMAN, H.H., *Am. Int. Med. 29* (1947), 22.
4. STEINBROCKER, O., *Ann. Phys. Med. Rehab. 49* (1968), 388.
5. GOLDING, D.N., *Ann. Rheum. Dis. 29* (1970), 10.
6. KOZIN, F., McCARTY, D.L., SIMS, J. and GENANT, H., *Am. J. Med. 60* (1976), 321.
7. BRIDGMAN, J.F., *Ann. Rheum. Dis. 31* (1972), 69.
8. WEISS, J.J., THOMPSON, G.R. and WOODBURY, D., *Mech. Med. 72* (1973), 771.
9. HART, F.D., 'Shoulder pain' in *French's Dictionary of Differential Diagnosis* (John Wright, Bristol, 11th edn, 1979), 723–6.

Chapter 7

1. ANSELL, B., 'Chronic Arthritis in Childhood' (Heberden Oration), in *Ann Rheum. Dis. 37* (1978), 107.
2. WYKE, B. 'Neurological aspects of low back pain' in *The Lumbar Spine and Back Pain*, ed. M.I.V. Jayson (Pitman Medical, London, 1976).

Chapter 8

1. ANSELL, B., *Juvenile Spondylitis and Related Disorders in Ankylosing Spondylitis*, ed. J.M.H. Moll (Churchill Livingstone, Edinburgh and London, 1980), 120.
2. MACNAB, I., *Backache* (Williams and Wilkins, Baltimore, 1977).

Chapter 9

1. GARROD, A.B., *Nature and Treatment of Gout and Rheumatic Gout* (Walton & Maberly, London, 1859).
2. HUTCHINSON, J., 'The Relation of Certain Diseases of the Eye to Gout', Bowman Lecture, *Lancet 2* (1884), 978.
3. HORTON, B.T., MAGATH, T.B. and BROWN, G.E., *Annals of Internal Medicine 53* (1934), 400.
4. BARBER, H.S., *Annals of Rheumatic Diseases 16* (1957), 230.
5. ANSELL, B.M. and BYWATERS, E.G.L., 'Diagnosis of Probable Still's Disease and Its Outcome', *Annals of Rheumatic Diseases 21* (1962), 253–61.

Chapter 10

1. AKHTAR, A.J., BROE, G.A., CROSBIE, A. et al, *Age and Ageing 2* (1973), 102.
2. KELLGREN, J.H. and MOORE, R., *Brit. Med. J. 1* (1952), 181.
3. FOX, R.A., *Europ. J. Rheum. and Inflam. 5* (1982), 285.
4. OKA, M., KYTILA, J., *Acta. Rheum. Scand. 3* (1957), 249.
5. *National Health Formulary*, British Medical Assn. and Pharm. Soc. of Great Britain. No. 1 (1981), 7.
6. BRAVERMAN, A.M., *Europ. J. Rheum. and Inflam. 5* (1981), 289.
7. INMAN, W.H., *Brit. Med. J. 1* (1977), 1500.
8. COOKE, P. and THOMSON, M.R., *Proc. Brit. Soc. Gastro-ent.* (1981), Abs. from *Gut 22(5)* (1981), A430 F.
9. GLEESON, M.H., *Europ. J. Rheum. and Inflam. 2* (1981).

Chapter 11

1. ANSELL, B.A., 'Chronic Arthritis in Childhood' (Heberden Oration), *Ann. Rheum. Dis. 37* (1978), 107.

Chapter 13

1. BARBER, H.S., 'Myalgic Syndrome with Corticosteroid Effects: Polymyalgia Rheumatica', *Ann. Rheum. Dis. 16* (1957), 230.
2. HAMRIN, B., 'Polymyalgia arteritica', *Acta. Med. Scand. Supp. 1* (1972), 533.
3. MYLES, A.B., 'Polymyalgia Rheumatica and Giant Cell Arteritis: a seven year survey', *Rheum. and Rehab. 14* (1975), 231.
4. HART, F.D., 'Visual complications of polymyalgia rheumatica (polymyalgia arteritica)', *Practitioner 215* (1975), 763.

Chapter 17

1. COPEMAN, W.S.C. in *Textbook of the Rheumatic Diseases,* ed. W.S.C. Copeman (E. & S. Livingstone, Edinburgh, 1st edn, 1948), 307.
2. STOCKMAN, R., *Rheumatism and Arthritis* (Green, Edinburgh, 1920).
3. COPEMAN, W.S.C. and ACKERMAN, W.L., *Quart. J. Med. 13* (1944), 37.
4. SMYTHE, H.A. in *Textbook of Rheumatology*, ed. Kelley, Harris, Ruddy and Sledge (W.B. Saunders, Philadelphia, 1981), 485.
5. KELLGREN, J.H. in Copeman's *Textbook of the Rheumatic Diseases*, ed. J.T. Scott (Churchill Livingstone, Edinburgh, 5th edn, 1978), 67.

Chapter 18

1. SZASZ, T.S., *Pain and Pleasure* (Basic Books Inc., New York, 2nd edn, 1975).

Chapter 21

1. CARUSO, I. and BIANCHI PORRO, G., *Brit. Med. J. 280* (1980), 75.
2. LANZA, F.L. et al., *Dig. Dis. and Sci. 24* (1979), 823.
3. DOUTHWAITE, A.H. and LINTOTT, G.A.M., *Brit. Med. J. 2* (1938), 1222.
4. HOFTIEZER, J.W. et al., *Lancet 2* (1980), 609.
5. GROSSMAN, M.I., MATSUMOTO, K.K. and LICHTER, R.J., *Gastroenterology 40* (1961), 383.
6. COOKE, A.R. and GOULSTON, K., *Brit. Med. J. 3* (1969), 330.
7. COOKE, A.R. and GOULSTON, K., *Brit. Med. J. 4* (1968), 664.

8. BOUCHER, I.A.D. and WILLIAMS, H.S., *Lancet 1* (1969), 178.

9. PLOTZ, P.A. in *Textbook of Rheumatology*, ed. Kelly et al., (W.B. Saunders, Philadelphia 1981), 752.

10. BATTERMAN, R.C., *N. Eng. J. Med. 258* (1958), 213.

11. CRONK, G.A., *N. Eng. J. Med. 258* (1958), 219.

12. LINNOKA, M., LEHTOLA, J., *Int. J. Clin. Pharm & BIOpharm. 15* (1977), 61.

13. SPIRO, H.M. in INGELFINGER, F.J., *Controversy in Internal Medicine II*, (W.B. Saunders, Philadelphia, 1974).

14. LEVY, M., *New. Eng. J. Med. 290* (1974), 1158.

15. FAMAEY, J.P. et al., *Ann. Int Med. 87* (1977), 676.

17. WELCH, R.W., BENTCH, H.L. and HARRIS, S.C., *Gastroenterology 74* (1978), 459.

Chapter 24

1. NEWTON, P., SHARP, J. and BARNES, K.L., 'Bone and Joint Tuberculosis in Greater Manchester, 1969–1979', *Ann. Rheum. Dis 41* (1981), 1.

2. HALSEY, J.P., REEBACK, J.S. and BARNES, C.G., 'A Decade of Skeletal Tuberculosis', *Ann. Rheum. Dis. 41* (1982), 7.

Chapter 25

1. KELLGREN, J.H. and MOORE, R., Generalised Osteoarthritis in Heberden's Nodes', *Brit. Med. J. 1* (1952), 181.

Chapter 26

1. Empire Rheumatism Council, *Ann. Rheum. Dis 19* (1960), 95; *20* (1961), 315.

Chapter 28

1. HART, F.D. (ed.), *Drug Treatment of the Rheumatic Diseases* (Adis Press, Auckland, 2nd edn, 1982).

2. MAINI, R.N. and BERRY, H. (eds), *Modulation of Auto-immunity and Disease: the penicillamine experience* (Praeden, Eastbourne and New York, 1981).

Chapter 29

1. BOARDMAN, P.L. and HART, F.D., *Brit. Med. J. 4* (1967), 264.

2. SKJELBRED, P., ALSUM, B. and LOKKEN, P., *Europ. J. Clin. Pharm. 12* (1977), 257.

3. CARUSO, I. and PORRO, G.B., *Brit. Med. J. 280* (1980), 75.

4. HART, F.D., *Drug Treatment of the Rheumatic Diseases* (Adis Press, Auckland, 2nd edn, 1982), 38.

5. LANZA, F.L. et al., *Dig. Dis. and Sci. 24* (1979), 823.

6. HART, op. cit., 43.

7. BABER, N. et al., *Ann. Rheum. Dis. 38* (1979), 128.

8. ORME, M. et al., *Scand. J. Rheum. Supp. 39* (1981) 19.

9. HUSKISSON, E.C. et al., *Brit. Med. J. 1* (1976), 1048.

Chapter 30

1. HAYNES, R.C., Jr and MURAD, F. in *The Pharmacological Basis of Therapeutics*, ed. A.G. Gilman, L.S. Goodman and A. Gilman (Macmillan, New York, 6th edn, 1980), 1466.

2. CHRISTIAN, C.C., 'Systemic Lupus Erythematosus' in *Drug Treatment of the Rheumatic Diseases*, ed. F. D. Hart (Adis Press, Auckland, 2nd edn, 1982), 159.
3. ISENBERG, D.A., MORROW, W.J.W. and SNAITH, M.L., 'Methylprednisolone Therapy in the Treatment of Systemic Lupus Erythematosus, *Ann. Rheum. Dis. 41* (1982), 347–51.

Chapter 33

1. ROBINSON, W.D. in *Textbook of Rheumatology*, ed. W.N. Kelley et al., (W.B. Saunders, Philadelphia, 1981), 337.
2. BAUER, W., *J.A.M.A. 104* (1935), 1.
3. BAYLES, T.B., RICHARDSON, H. and HALL, F.C., *New Eng. J. Med. 299* (1943), 319.
4. *Diet in Arthritis* (The American Arthritis Foundation, Atlanta).
5. PARKE, A.L. and HUGHES, G.R.V., *Brit. Med. J. 282* (1981), 2027.
6. HUSKISSON, E.C. and HART, F.D., *Joint Disease* (John Wright, Bristol, 3rd edn, 1978), 24.

Useful Addresses

Arthritis Care (The British Rheumatism
and Arthritis Association)
6 Grosvenor Crescent
London SW1X 7ER

The Arthritis and Rheumatism Council
for Research
41 Eagle Street
London WC1R 4AR

The Back Pain Association
31–3 Park Road
Teddington
Middlesex MX TW11 OAB

The British League Against Rheumatism
c/o The Arthritis and Rheumatism
Council for Research (above)

The British Red Cross Society
9 Grosvenor Crescent
London SW1X 7EG
(for coordination and information)

The Disabled Living Foundation
346 Kensington High Street
London W14 8NS

The Horder Centre For Arthritics
Crowborough
Sussex TN6 1XP
(for research and information)

The Royal Association for Disability
and Rehabilitation
25 Mortimer Street
London W1N 8AB

The Scottish Council on Disability
18–19 Claremont Crescent
Edinburgh EH7 4QD
(for information and aids)

AUSTRALIA

The Australian Arthritis and
Rheumatism Foundation
12th Floor
291 George Street
Sydney
NSW 2000

The Australian Association of
Occupational Therapists
11 Grose Street
Camperdown
NSW 2050

The Australian Association of Physical
and Rehabilitation Medicine
c/o Multiple Sclerosis Society of
Victoria
616 Riversdale Road
Camberwell
Victoria 3124

The Australian College of
Rehabilitation Medicine
PO Box 851
Ryde
NSW 2112

The Australian Orthopaedic
Association
299–31 Macquaire Street
Sydney
NSW 2000

The Australian Rheumatism
Association
(doctors only – communicate via The
Australian Arthritis and Rheumatism
Foundation, above)

The Lupus Society
23 Marks Street
Naremburn
NSW 2065

The Parents of Arthritic Children
5 Owen Street
Lindfield
NSW 2070

Acknowledgements

The authorand publishers are grateful to the Westminster Hospital Medical School Department of Medical Illustration and Teaching Services and especially to Keith Duguid, FRPS, FBIPP, AIMBI, Head of the Department, for their assistance in providing the following photographs: Figures, 3, 6, 7, 9, 10, 11, 24, 31, 35, 43, 57, 58, 62, 64, 65, 66, 67, 68, 69a–d, 70, 73, 74, 76, 80a–95a.

We should also like to thank Dr Peter Fowler for permission to reproduce Figure 32 and Dr S.P. Liyanage for Figure 59. All other photographs are supplied by the author.

The table on page 62 is based on 'Back Pain' in *French's Index of Differential Diagnosis*, ed. F. Dudley Hart (John Wright, Bristol, 11th edn, 1979) page 86, and is reproduced by kind permission of the publishers.

The diagrams are by David Gifford.

Index

Figures in italics refer to illustrations.